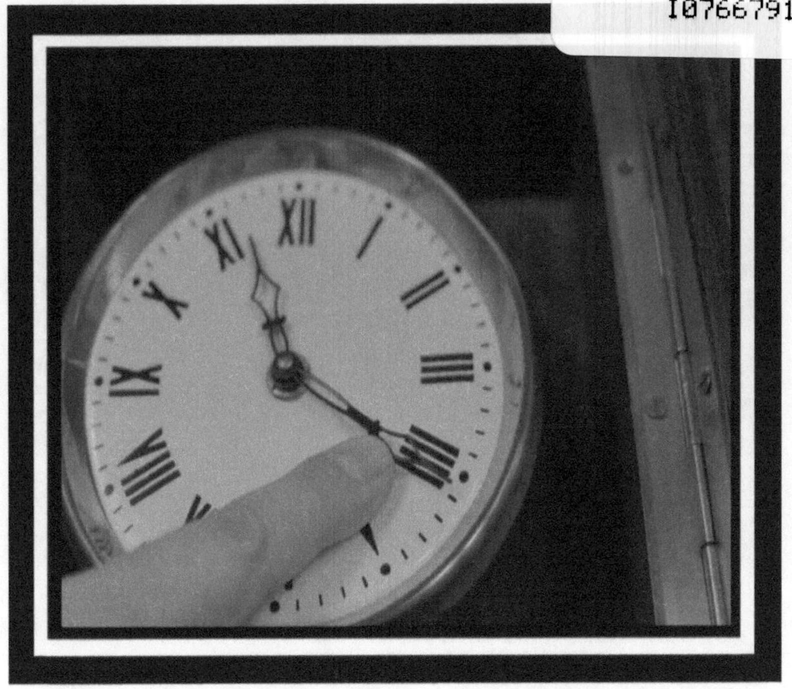

Holdin' Back the Years!

Inexpensive Spa at Home Tips with Easy

Do-it-Yourself Recipes for Anti-Aging

By

Tasher

Contributions from

Latica Mirjanic, MA Psych

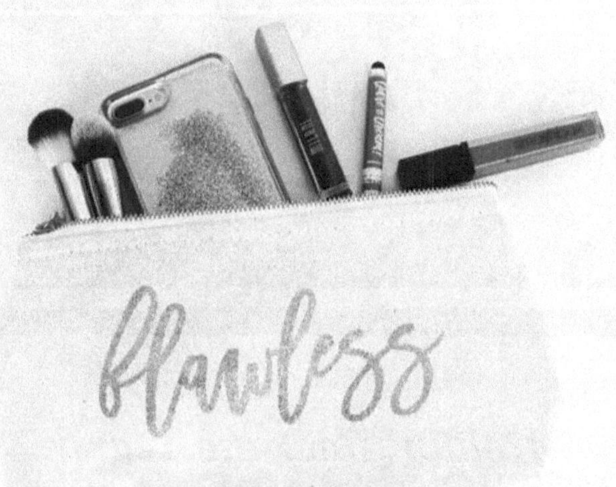

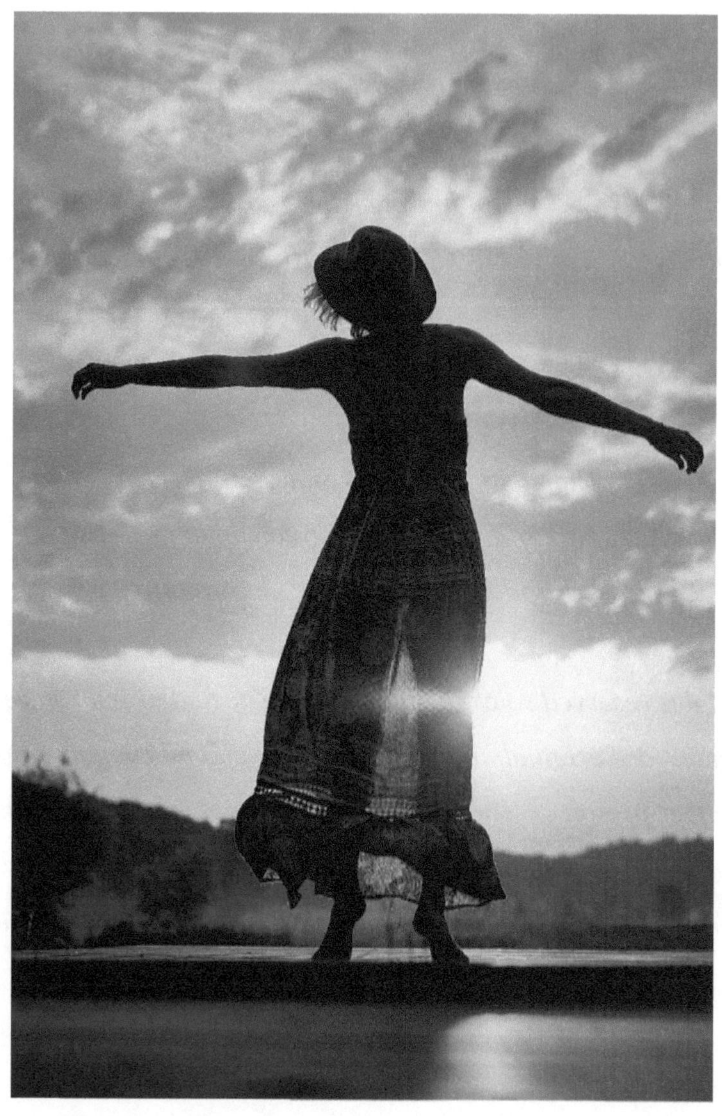

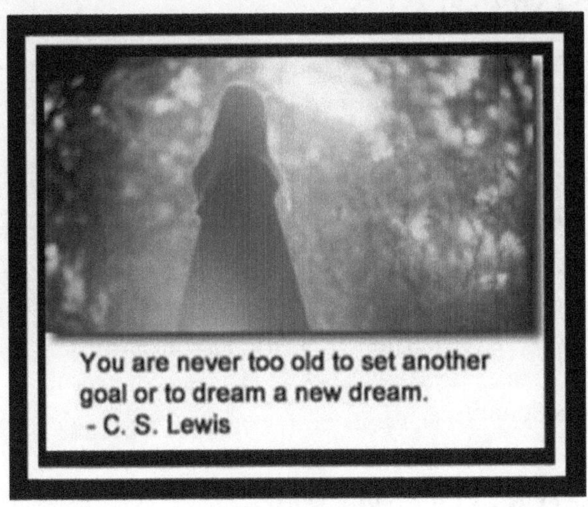

Table of Contents

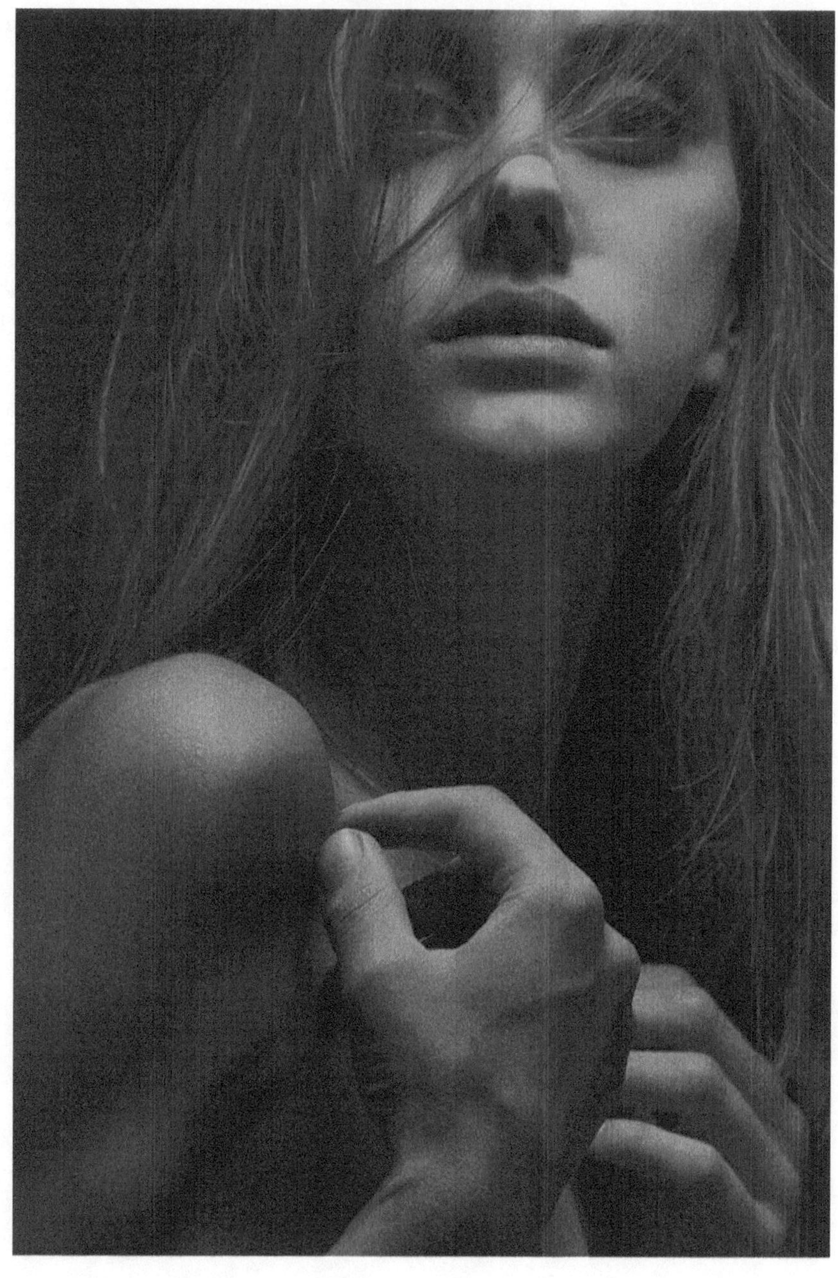

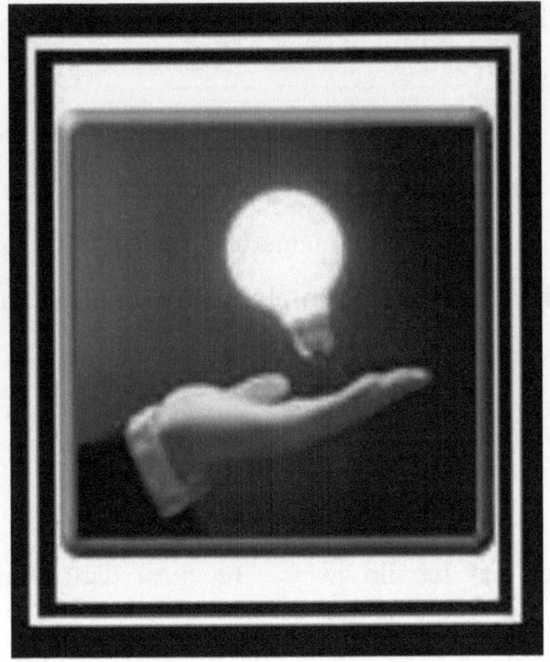

Dedication

To my children and grandchildren, thank you for all your love and support. Having dyslexia, I was fearful of writing books even though I always enjoyed telling stories… With your love and support, I am now on my fourth book! You always gave me the strength to take each step forward, especially in the days during and after the divorce. I saw you believed and supported me when I had moments of doubting myself. Thank you for always being there for me. Thank you for being the best cheerleaders any person could ever hope to have! Always remember, "I love you to the moon and back to infinity, now and forever. You are the loves of my life and my reason for being!"

The website Divorced and Scared NO More was online from 2012 until 2019. The site included many topics such as etiquette, co-parenting, finances… After numerous requests, we added things people could do to pamper themselves. The members quickly started sharing their beauty secrets. These smart and savvy newly single people wanted to look even more fantastic now than they did when they were married! Being on the market again, they were determined to put their best foot forward while making the EX see what a beautiful gem they let slip away. But those darn finances or lack thereof got in the way. In this book, I have compiled most of the information shared on the website, Facebook page, Twitter, along with my family secrets, plus a few I have found on my own.

I also dedicated this book to all of you who have decided to become frugal for whatever reason. Being frugal is fun and can become a sport to see how much you can save to have extra cash to spend on other fun things, or put a little more cushion in your bank account! Instead of letting the lemons of time age you, turn them into a beauty treatment. Use those lemons to hold back the signs of time. While doing so, you can also treat yourself to a zesty lemon sorbet while you are relaxing at your very own home spa!

Tasher

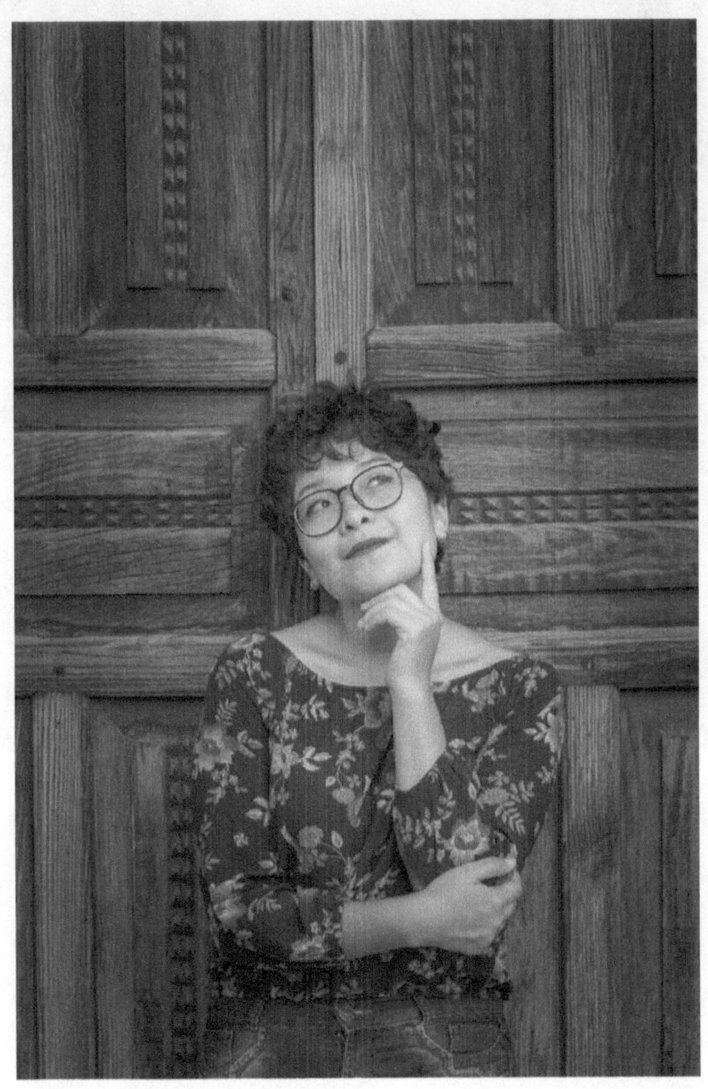

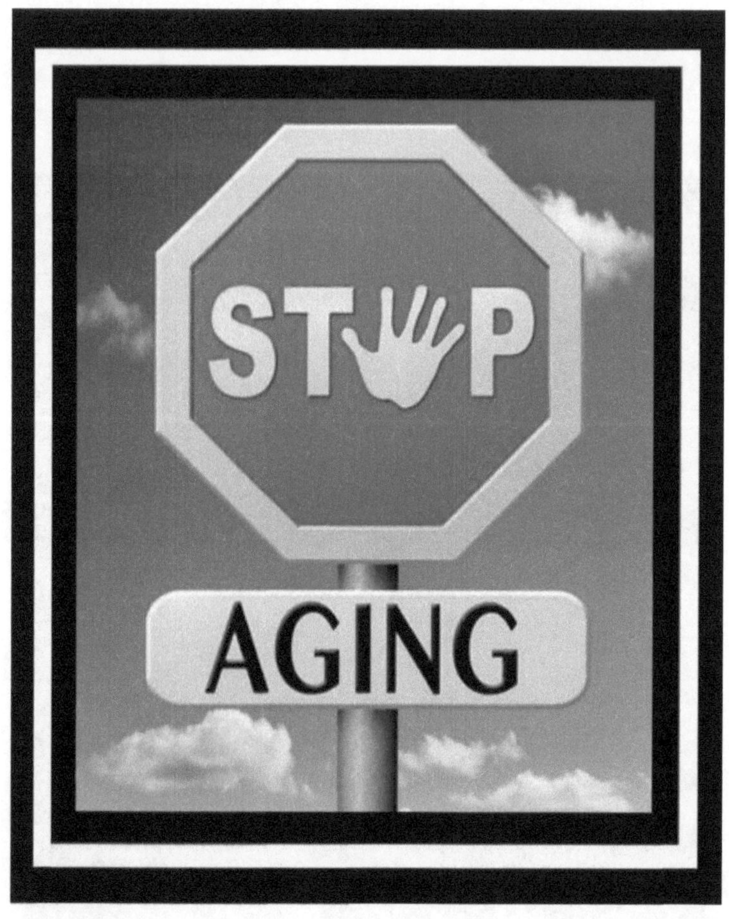

STOP
AGING

Introduction to Health and Beauty Care

Ever wanted to make do-it-yourself recipes for face creams or anti-wrinkle cream that really would work, but you never knew how? Do it yourself skin creams and face masks on a tight budget using everyday ingredients. Many members of the Divorced and Scared NO More website, Facebook, Twitter, along with my family and friends, have not only found things that work they are thrilled to share them with you. In this book, you will find easy do-it-yourself recipes for anti-aging, wrinkle, and face creams as well as various other at-home treatments. You don't have to be a rocket scientist or turn your kitchen into a laboratory to make these fun formulas that can save your skin and money at the same time. Not sure about you but that's my kind of multi-tasking!

Always remember to perform a patch test to check for allergies when you are trying any new ingredient or beauty product. Then to be on the safe side, wait 24 hours to make sure you don't have any redness, swelling or itchiness. Soon you will be asking yourself, "What is it about mixing up a homemade face mask that makes it so much fun, and why didn't I start sooner?" You will find yourself experimenting with these recipes and tweaking the ones you like making them perfect for your skin and hair to increase your youthful glow.

Don't be afraid to try making homemade face masks and scrubs, as you will see; it is relatively simple. Why pay for expensive store-bought face mask when many of the necessary ingredients required are probably in your house today to make beauty treatments, for free or only cost pennies?

Generation to Generations

I am sure your family is just like mine and have many beauty secrets that have been handed down over the years. The first one I learned was during my first pregnancy. Every time an older female in my family saw me, with a raised eyebrow, asked if I was using my baby oil????? The family secret is to rub baby oil all over your body at least twice a day while pregnant to reduce getting stretch marks. I will admit during the first pregnancy; I did it just out of love and respect for my elders. I never realized how well it worked until a few of my friends and I were out shopping for bathing suits. I was shocked to see the stretch marks they had. No female in my family had those pesky little lines. I made sure during my other pregnancies; I used the baby oil three times a day. Over the years, I have come up with a beauty oil for daily use to hold back the years. It does not have any baby oil in it, but instead, it's base is my homemade monoi oil with some essential oils. Before you ask yes, I will share the recipe for my homemade monoi oil later in the book. Using the oil daily and building one day upon the last is what works. You can't have years of neglect then soak yourself in some miracle cream or lotion and expect anything to happen. What all those miracle creams and lotions do is make your money disappear. It is a process of one day built upon the last, and it's just that simple. I am now over 50, the numbers on my scale have gone up and down, and I am proud to say I still do not have any stretch marks.

Here are a few of the most popular secrets from the DASNM (Divorced and Scared NO More) mothers/grandmothers to you.

- Steam your face weekly and follow with a hydrating mask.

- Other than preventing a unibrow or a wild hair here and there, don't touch those brows! As we age, our hair thins, plus the back half of your eyebrows seem to disappear. Instead, use castor oil mixed with a few drops of rosemary on your brows every other day. After you see the results, I bet you will start believing in the power of natural products. The earlier you start (and stick with it) the better your brows will be for the rest of your life

- Homemade body mask. Mix ground Turmeric, ground Oatmeal, Honey, a bit of Milk, Lemon juice, flour and rosewater into a thick paste. Apply the mixture all over your body in circular motions to exfoliate. Leave it on for 15-20 minutes then shower with a loofah. Making sure to wash off the mask in a circular motion.

- Wash and moisturize your face in the morning and before going to bed. Doing so helps prevent pimples, plus your skin will last longer and look younger. If you are young, you may be questioning my "last longer" comment. As we age, our skin gets thinner paler, translucent, and at some point, you will look at yourself and say I miss my skin.

- The real trick with moisturizer is the application technique, especially when applying it to the delicate skin around your eyes. Dot the moisturizer on and gently smooth it out in an upward motion with your middle or ring finger. Do not ever rub hard or tug on your skin; doing so can encourage wrinkles.

- Exfoliate your entire body several times a week.

- Use egg whites as a face mask; it's great for tightening pores.

- Use tea tree oil on your hair and face. Tea tree oil has been used for a very long time to help with acne problems. Did you know it also can protect against head lice? Those little critters are repelled by tea tree oil. The scent is very potent; remember a little goes a very long way.

- It is always best to look fresh, avoid a heavy hand. Makeup applied lightly will give you a refreshed younger look. Unless you are going to a children's party as the entertainer you don't want to look like a clown, do you?

- There is no 'best' when it comes to beauty. But there is a key to tapping into the real beauty that people can see blocks away; it is **CONFIDENCE!** Have you ever witnessed a woman with a few extra pounds, entering a room and all heads turn to her with smiles? You can feel the place begin to fill with happiness with each step she takes into the room. A few moments later, a thin, sad-looking woman enters, and no one even notices she is there?

- If you want your hair a few shades lighter but do not want to put any dye in your hair. Mix fresh-squeezed lemon juice with water and liberally apply on your hair. Then have fun in the sun while your hair naturally air dries. Make sure to wear sunscreen while frolic in the sun, Wash the lemon water cocktail completely out of your hair after about an hour. The citric acid found in lemons exposed to UV rays from the sun will have a lightning effect on the hair. DO NOT attempt this if you have chemically treated hair of any type because it will create a very undesirable result.

- Need to relax your muscles. and soothe blister pain for sore, aching feet, prepare a foot bath containing: 1-part water, 1-part oatmeal, 1-part vinegar 1-part Aloe Vera and 1-part Epsom salts. Soak your feet for at least 30 minutes then dry them off. Follow by elevating the feet above your heart level for another 30 minutes.

- Cut the Aloe leaf Generously apply Aloe Vera to cool a sunburn. You can cut the leaf open and apply the gel from inside or if you prefer there are many over the counter Alee gels you can buy. But please make sure you are getting 100% Alee or as close as possible. Remember it is always good to read the labels

- To reduce or avoid bladder leakage start these suggestions when you are young. Your older self will thank you! Following these suggestions should help anyone of any age keep or regain some control and not have leakage.

- o When you feel the urge to go to the restroom, instead wait and hold the urine for 5 to 10 minutes. Each time you feel the urge slowly increase the holding time until you get to 30 minutes. Do at least one 30-minute hold a day.

- o A supplement that works well for many women is AZO Bladder Control with Go-Less (with or without Weight Management). "Azo products are available online at AzoProducts.com

- Ladies start doing your Kegel exercises whenever you are at a stop sign or stoplight.

  - o How to do Kegel exercises:

    - Tighten your pelvic floor muscles. Hold tight and count to 8.
    - Relax the muscles and count to 10.
    - Repeat 10 times
    - Breathe deeply and relax your body when you are doing these exercises. Make sure you are not tightening your stomach, thigh, buttock, or chest muscles.

- Use rag rollers for hair that never wants to stay curled. Wet your hair and roll it up in rags. Sleep with your rag rollers in place while your hair dries overnight. In the morning, you have super curly hair.

- Make homemade hair masque from Honey, coconut oil. or mayonnaise. Apply any one of the three liberally and let it sit on your hair for 30 to 60 minutes then wash out of your hair.

- Hydrating lip tint, A&D ointment, or balm before bed is excellent for helping nourish lips while you sleep. Plus, you never know when a firefighter may have to come in and rescue you. The lip tint will make you look pretty while you sleep.

- Sleep on your back to avoid wrinkles and sleep lines from forming on both the face and chest.

- Lack of sleep will show in your face via puffy eyes and wrinkles, so get your 7 to 8 hours sleep a night.

- Weekly rinse your hair with a glass of half vinegar and half water. The rinse can make your hair feel silky soft.

Important Points to Remember Before You Begin

- Always wash your hands before starting a DIY recipe. Making beauty care products is just like food; you don't want to contaminate it.

- Try to use dark glass containers. They protect the potency of the product you are making. Plastic or light have horrible effects on essential oils!

- Never turn your stove temperature over medium heat while making your potions because the heat can affect the quality and potency of your DIY products. Always use the minimum amount of heat to keep your oils potent.

- Add essential oils at the very end. The heat renders them ineffective. Sometimes with creams/salves/balms, I will let them cool completely, add essential oils, then slowly mix in the creams/salve/balm. It gives your salves/balms a creamier consistency.

- Most of all, have fun. If you can cook or you can at least follow a recipe, then you can make fantastic beauty care products.

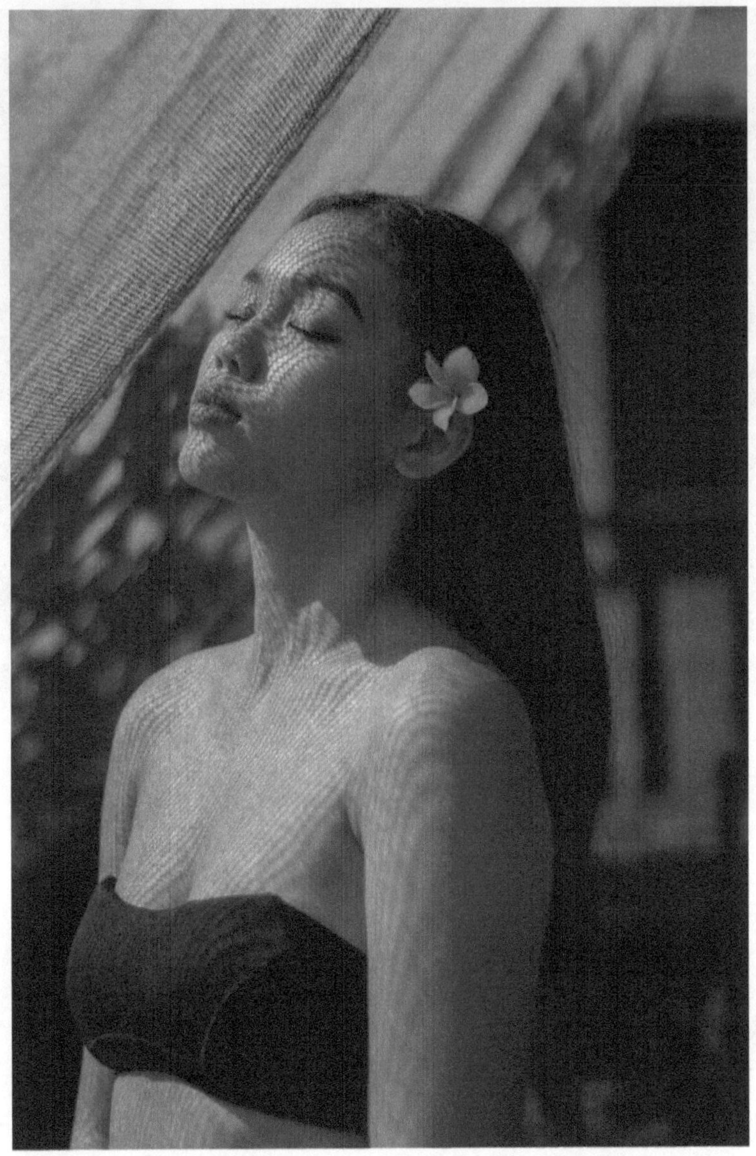

Holdin' Back the Years!

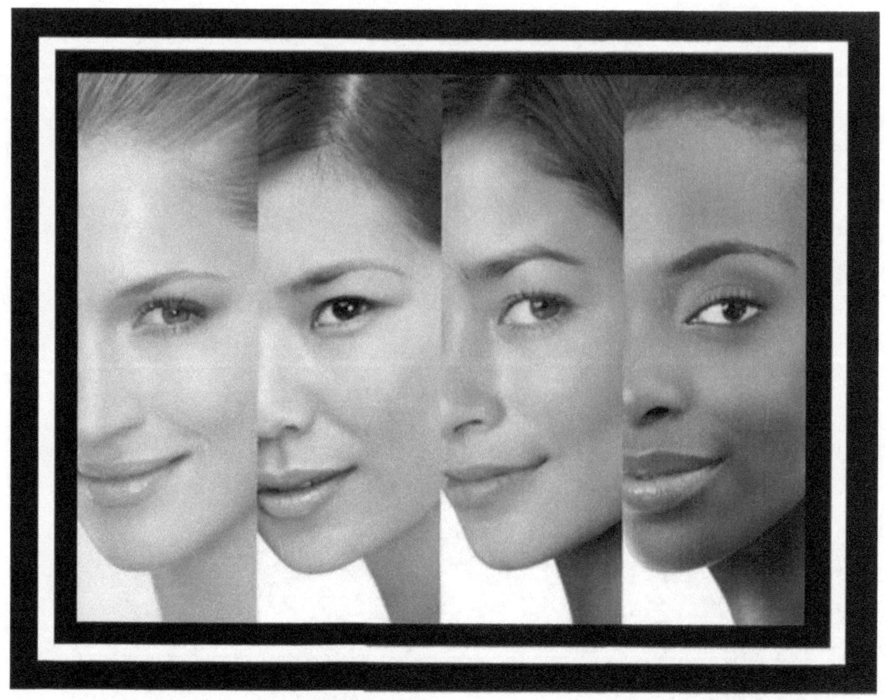

Chapter 1

Cashmere Care for Skin

Who needs Botox when you have bananas? When you want a quick way to give your skin, some TLC a banana is a quick all-natural homemade facial mask. It is a fast way to moisturizes your skin, plus it will look and feel softer. Mash up a medium-sized ripe banana into a smooth paste, apply to your face and neck. Leave the mask on for 10-15 minutes. Wash off with a steaming hot washcloth. Run the washcloth under warm water, squeeze out the excess water and then press on your face for a full minute. Now gently wash off the mask in a circular motion. Washcloths are brilliant for exfoliating. The final phase is to rinse your face with cold water and pat dry. Wasn't that easy? Now you have done your first DIY beauty treatment. Let's get our caldrons out and start cookin or should I say mixin up some more fun masks to try! Wink wink!

Facial Masks

Apple Carrot Facial Mask

If you have acne-prone skin, the apple carrot mask can help reduce breakouts.

Directions:

Squeeze the juice out of an Apple

Cook and mash a big Carrot.

Mix Carrot with Apple juice. Add 2-3 tbs. of Honey until you get a light paste.

Smooth over skin in a circular motion then let it sit for 10 minutes.

Rinse off with cold water.

Glowing Facial Mask

Ingredients:

1 tbsp. Rose Clay Powder

1 tbsp. Mashed Avocado

Directions:

Add water until you get a silky mask

Mix well and put on the face for 20 minutes then rinse off.

Orange Yogurt Mask

Ingredients:

2 tsp. full-fat Greek Yogurt

Squeeze Lemon Juice

1 tbs. of Honey

Directions:

Mix well and smooth onto face. The sensation is both refreshing and relaxing. Leave on for 20 minutes and then rinse.

More Moisture / Clearer Skin / Fade Spots on Skin with Honey

Here's one to try, cut an orange in quarters, and add Honey to the top of the orange. Add a few drops of tea tree oil.

Rub on top all over your face in a circular motion. Take a little extra time on troubled areas.

Leave the mixture on for 10 minutes.

Rinse off with cold water

Full Body DIY Recipes for Homemade Skin-Care Treatments

It is pretty easy to duplicate some treatments found at upscale spas while keeping your hard-earned money in your bank account or pocket. Here are a few ideas I have seen.

Moisturize Your Skin

Ingredients:

2 ripe Bananas

2 ripe Papaya

1 cup Whipping Cream

Orange Essential Oil

Eucalyptus Essential Oil

Directions:

Place all the ingredients one at a time in a food processor, blending until you get a smooth and silky consistency. Apply all over your body (avoiding the eyes). Wrap yourself up using food storage wrap. After 10 minutes, take a warm shower.

Skin Balm

Ingredients:

2 teaspoons Olive Oil

1 teaspoon Shea Butter

4 drops Orange Essential Oil

Directions:

Mix shea butter and olive oil on low heat until they blend. Wait a few minutes then add the orange essential oil. Pour the mixture into a dark glass jar. Store in a cool, dry place.

DIY Anti-Aging for under $1

Are you starting to notice that so many of the ingredients you need are already in your home? Here are a few beauty potions that will cost you under $1.

Cherry Wrinkle Blaster

Ingredients:

Zest of freshly squeezed Lemon

4 tablespoons Honey

Ripe Avocado

Directions:

Combine the ingredients. Apply the mixture to the problem area. Leave for 15 minutes and rinse with warm water. Repeat a few times a week.

Egg Wash for Facial

Whip the Egg Whites until frothy. Apply to face and leave on for 30 minutes. Rinse with cold water and apply your usual face cream.

Olive Oil

Apply Olive Oil on your face and take a warm shower. If the oil is on your skin too long, it could clog your pores so after you get out of the shower to remove the oil from your face with makeup remover pads. Finally, rinse your face with cold water and apply your usual face cream.

Keep those Coffee Grounds

Many of us love a nice cup of coffee to get us going in the morning. Did you know that there are lots of uses for the leftover grounds? Coffee grounds have been used for everything from beauty tricks to odor reducers, pest repellents, and the list goes on and on. Here are a couple of ideas to get you started.

Facial Exfoliating Mask

Mix 2 tablespoons of Coffee Grounds with 1 teaspoon Coconut Oil. Apply on your face in a circular motion and leave on for 10 minutes. Rinse with warm water.

Skin Softener

Make a body scrub equal parts Coffee Grounds and Almond Oil. Gently massage it all over your body, shower, rinse, and feel your fantastic soft silky skin.

A Solution for Crepey Skin

Almost everyone will experience having crepey skin. The texture of the skin becomes like that of an elephant, with a crepe paper texture. I have to admit when I first started showing signs of crepey skin, it did look weird and scary. I felt it was making me look OLD. Yikes, and it was in my decollete' to boot. The area of my body that took years to get looking just right and now crepey skin had moved in. Many people had told me over the years there is one good part about crepey skin and that is it's treatable.

There are many lotions, potions, and home remedies for crepey skin. Please use your common sense when trying any home remedy. Remember, as previously stated, there are no "miracle cures" or "magic remedies" that are going to make anything vanish completely, especially not overnight! If you have any questions about any skincare products, please consult your healthcare provider.

Moisture is a must to wake up the dead cells. Use a cream or lotion with antioxidants, making sure it also has Vitamin A, C and E. Regular use of sunscreens and lotions will help you avoid crepey skin. You can also add copper peptides, Retin- A, Glycolic acid, and Hyaluronic acid.

Here are some of the home remedies you can try to get rid of your crepey skin.

1. Massage skin wherever there is crepey skin daily. Do not skip one day!

2. Moisturize as much as you can because the lack of moisture is the key reasons behind the crepey skin. You must moisturize your body from head to toe, making sure to massage it in.

3. Exfoliate -- You might not have known that manual exfoliation also helps to trigger elastin and collagen production in the body.

4. Exercise is one of the best home remedies for crepey skin. The lack of regular exercise is also one of the reasons behind the crepey skin. Regular exercise will bring back the flexibility in your muscles and promote the increase in the level of Elastin and Collagen.

Add a daily dose of Collagen Peptide to your coffee or juice. Collagen is the most abundant protein in the body, ensuring the health and vitality of your skin, hair, tendons, cartilage, bones, and joints. Natural peptides are highly bio-available, digestible, and soluble in cold or hot liquids. Run a cool-mist humidifier in your bedroom at night. People living in a dry climate will find adding humidity to the room will be especially helpful in preventing wrinkles and getting moisture in your skin.

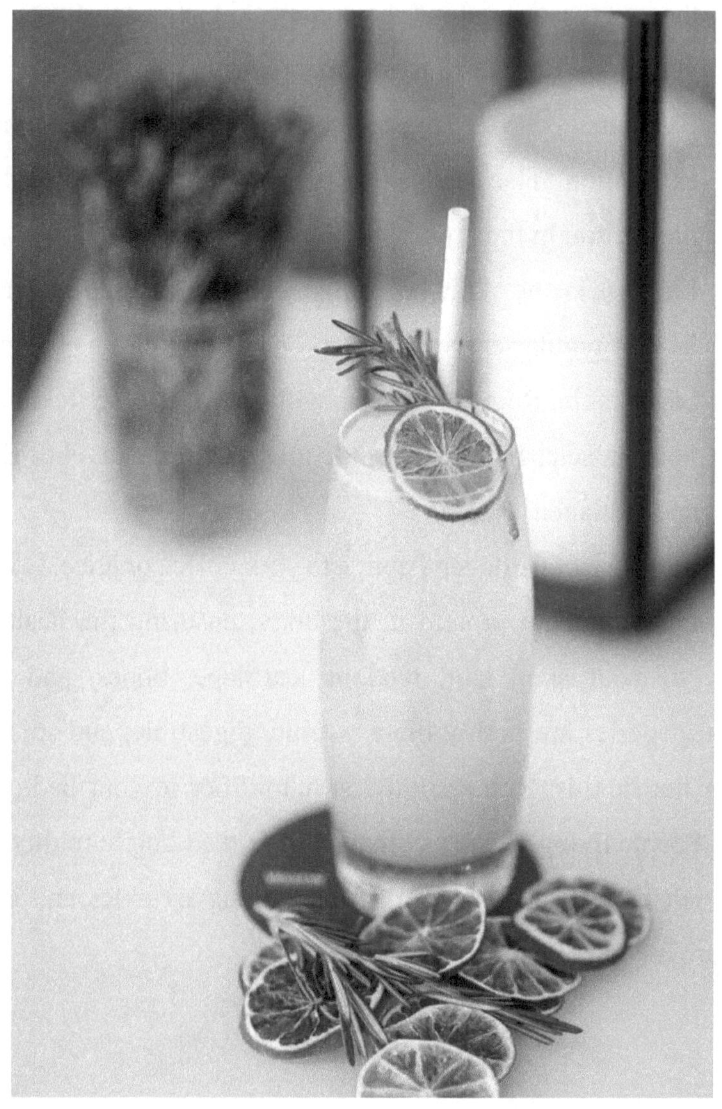

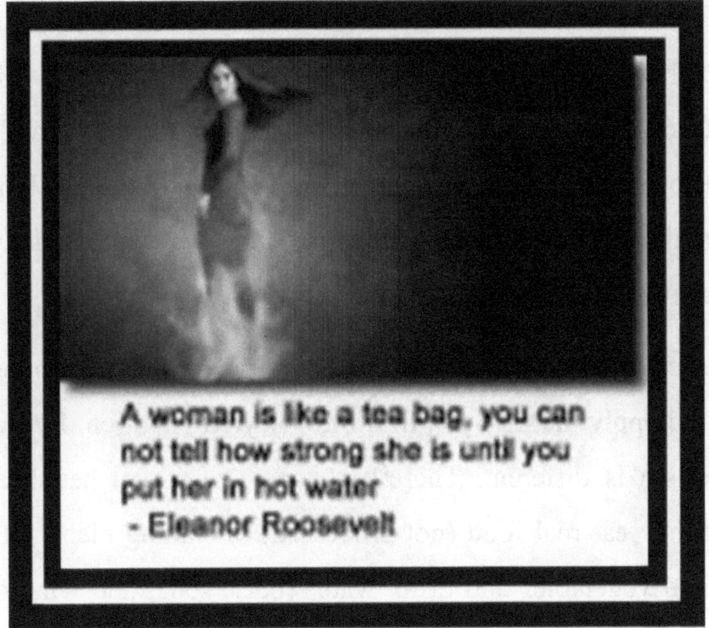

Chapter 2

Common Sense Health Tips

This chapter is excerpted from the Divorced and Scared
NO More series book 2 Practical Advice for the Newly
Divorced __by Tasher

The upset, and the strain of any significant life-altering event can leave you emotional and physical health at risk. (For more information regarding rebuilding your life after the effects of divorce, see the first book in the DASNM series, *Divorced and Scared No More: Emotional Support for the Newly Divorced.*)

After a divorce, for example, many tend not to have the best eating habits, the results become displayed on their waistlines. Making positive changes in eating habits will make you feel better and more energetic. You are going through an emotional wringer, dealing with some major life adjustments. Aid your recovery by making daily time for activities you find soothing and relaxing.

Listed below are tips that helped me, but please feel free to take the ideas and apply them as you deem fit for your situation. Everyone's metabolism is different. There's no one-size-fits-all health advice except this: eat real food (not processed), including plenty of fresh fruits and vegetables and drink water (beer, soda, and wine do not count as water, and they will seriously affect your mood). Start reading the labels of anything you put in your body, and if there are ingredients you cannot pronounce, it's safe to assume it's probably not healthy or right for you. No potion, drug, vitamin, or health routine will make you feel 100 percent, but with each step in the right direction, you will start feeling better.

Finally, you will feel better and see good results if you try some exercise, meditation, and daily spiritual growth. Consult your physician or other healthcare professional before starting any of the tips or any other suggestions in this book.

Start Today with the Basics

- **Don't skip meals, especially breakfast:** I noticed that when I skipped meals, I became more tired and irritable. Irritability does not help when you are already trying to change your life's routine. I started eating a healthy breakfast full of fiber and protein. Not only does your body get what is needed, but you will also feel full longer. Do not eat just because a clock says so. If you are not hungry, don't eat. Or have something simple like an apple for breakfast.

- **Choose to eat healthy foods first at every meal:** Who knew that eating foods in a particular order plays a role in your health? Start your meal with a small glass of water. Next, eat the healthy food on the plate, which might be a fresh green salad. After eating your healthy food, eat a small portion of the food you like best at the end of the meal. Only eat until you start to feel satisfied. End the meal on a positive note with the most pleasing taste. Instead of the "clean plate" club let's have a "leave a little for the angels" club?

- **Chew slowly and put your fork down after each bite:** Take time to chew and enjoy every bit of food during a meal. It is recommended you chew each piece of food five to fifty times, but really, who is counting? The more you chew, the longer the meal will last, and the longer it will take before you have to move on with ordinary life.

- **Throw out your bathroom scales:** Eat healthily and forget about the number on the scale. If your appearance is important to you, rely on measurements instead of weight. When you are stressed, your weight will fluctuate so much you might literally break the scale to pieces. Instead, sell the scale on eBay and buy yourself an adorable hat.

- **Take vitamins:** A good multivitamin, vitamin D, calcium, omega-3 fish oil, and Sam-e are my vitamins of choice. Don't forget vitamin D and omega-3s. They are mood stabilizers and help your energy stay at a level you can handle.

- **Walk away from the stress:** The parking space farthest away from the grocery store entrance became my parking place of choice. Climb the stairs instead of taking the elevator; at first, you may only do a floor or two, but soon you will be surprised how many stories you can go up without breaking a sweat. Set aside time for a thirty-minute walk each day. To increase my walking, I gave myself a rule: whenever I am on the phone, I walk while I talk. Every rule has an exception, and the exception here is answering a call while driving.

- **Start a workout routine:** Right now, you may want to lie in bed, but I promise once you start working out, you will see its benefits. Music like "Waka Waka (This Time for Africa)" by Shakira you can get up, start dancing, singing and moving. With exercise, you will feel better emotionally and physically, and your self-esteem, which is more than likely low right now, will increase. Train with weights to build strong muscles and bones. If you join a gym, you can also meet a new group of people at some of the classes they offer (keep this in mind when you're ready to start dating again; check out the third book in this series, *Divorced and Scared No More: Dating after Divorce—From Lemons to Zesty Lemon Sorbet* for pointers). You could also join a walking or running group but if you prefer, work out alone. Whatever you decide, get moving. The most important benefit of exercise is the increase in serotonin and endorphin levels. These "happy hormones" make you feel vibrant, instead of like a slug who doesn't care.

- **Get enough sleep:** The lack of sleep made me feel bad from the moment I woke up, a feeling that continued all day long. Did you know it getting enough sleep can reduce the risk of heart disease and diabetes?

- **Brush and floss your teeth twice daily:** Studies have shown good dental hygiene not only reduces the risk of the obvious dental problems but also reduces the risk of heart disease. Not to mention that it is hard to form a new group of friends if your breath and yellow teeth scare them away. Many healthcare professionals have found links between dental hygiene and chronic infection and almost every disease, including cancer.

Natural Headache Cures

Post-divorce, many people have commented they have an increase in the frequency of headaches. If you fall into this category, first contact your health care provider to see if there is any physical issue you should be addressing. I have high blood pressure, and with a headache, the first thing I do is check my blood pressure. If yours is high, seek professional help immediately. If the blood pressure is not high and after you've talked with your doctor, you may want to try some natural things I found to help with headaches. There are different types of headaches; take a few minutes to learn which type of a headache you may be having. For all kinds of headaches that are not related to blood pressure, start by drinking plenty of room-temperature water.

Tension Headaches are caused when the muscles that cover your skull contract. The pain goes from ear to ear and around the front of your head. Tension headaches are the most common type of headache members reported having. People usually get these because of stress or the lack of sleep. Here are some ways to combat tension headaches:

- Peppermint Oil: Rub the oil around your hairline. It will provide a cooling sensation (and a pleasant smell) and very often will relax the muscles and stop the contraction.

- Ginger Tea: Peel and either cut into small chunks or crush up about an inch of ginger root, adding it to boiling water. Ginger settles the stomach and reduces inflammation and worked for me about as well as taking an aspirin.

Cluster Headaches are the type of a headache in which pain emanates from one spot; many describe the pain like an ice pick stabbing into their head.

- Capsicum, Magnesium, or Melatonin: These are common natural remedies used to treat or reduce the symptoms of cluster headaches, according to WebMD.

Migraine Headaches bring severe throbbing pain and increased sensitivity to light and sound. Migraines can cause nausea for many. Researchers have noted this type of headache seems to run in families.

- Acupressure Massage: Place your finger in the depression between your first and second toe and press firmly for three to five minutes.

You should consult your physician or other healthcare professional before starting these natural headache tips or any other recommendations in this book. Do not take these suggestions if your physician or health care provider advises against it. I am not a professional; I am only offering information that has helped me personally. You should not rely on this information as a substitute for professional medical advice. If you have any concerns or questions about your health, you should always consult with a physician or other health-care professional.

Another Unsightly Bruise

You don't recall bumping into anything, but lately, you seem to be frequently bruising. Is this cause for concern? Bruises are the result of some type of trauma or injury to the skin that causes blood vessels to burst. Easy bruising can be frequent due to age and medication. Although most bruises are harmless and go away without treatment, easy bruising can sometimes be a sign of a severe problem. Some people — especially women — are more prone to bruising than others. As people, age skin becomes thinner and loses some of the protective fatty layers that help cushion blood vessels from injury. If you experience increased bruising, don't stop taking your medications. Talk to your doctor about your concerns.

Bruises usually go away on their own, but you can take steps to lessen the pain and reduce visibility. Here are a few things you can incorporate into your diet to assist the reducing age-related bruising.

Bromelain is derived from pineapples (actually the stem) and is a potent enzyme that has anti-inflammatory properties and plays a role in reducing bruising and swelling.

Quercetin is a plant flavonoid derived from fruits with anti-oxidant and anti-inflammatory properties. Foods with high amounts of quercetin include capers, apples, red onion, citrus fruit, and leafy green vegetables.

For hundreds of years, people have been using Arnica for minor injuries as well as bruising and swelling. The active ingredient in Arnica works deep down to reduce pain, swelling, and discoloration. Below is a recipe for some typical preparations for Arnica oil:

Used as an infusion (approximately 1 teaspoon dried herb in 1/2 cup water), tincture (approximately 1-part herb to 10 parts alcohol), oil (1-part dried herb in 5 parts plant oil) or mouth rinse (1-part tincture in 10 parts water) or ointment (1-part arnica oil to 4 or 5 parts base).3/4 cup oil infused with arnica (pour oil over 1-ounce dried herbs in a jar, shake daily for six weeks).

These homeopathic preparations of arnica are recommended for healthy adults. This treatment is not recommended for children, pregnant, or nursing women. Never apply anything to broken skin unless you are directed by your medical professional.

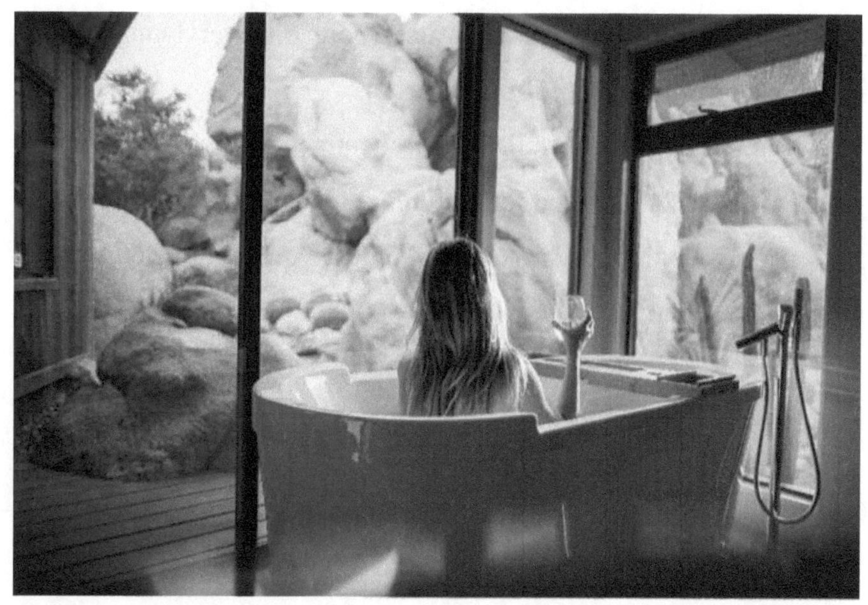

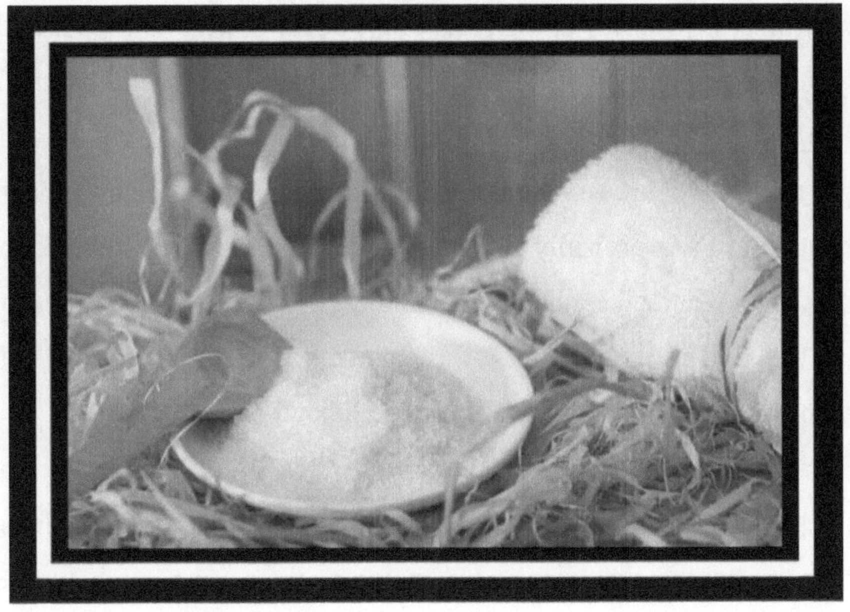

Chapter 3

A Splishin' and a Splashin'

I don't remember much about my life before moving to Fairbanks road. I was three years old when my father came home to announce he had purchased a farm at an auction and we were moving to the country to live on the farm. My Dad grew up on a farm, but my mother lived in a small town in Missouri. My mother was not quite prepared for the "new" house my Dad had bought at the auction. It was way out in the country on a dirt road (it's still a dirt road) between Linden and Fenton in Michigan. There was no indoor bathroom, but the over 100-year-old house did have an outhouse. I remember my father ripping parts of the house down to the studs and rebuilding it piece by piece. My love of baths started when I lived on Fairbanks road the day my Dad finished our indoor bathroom, and I got to cut a ribbon, celebrating we had a brand spanking new indoor bathroom! I was probably the most excited toddler to be able to use a "real potty" and take a bath in a bathtub again. Within a few days of my Dad finishing our indoor bathroom, the fire department visited our home because my mother was burning the outhouse down.

So as you can see as long as I can remember, I guess I have been a big proponent of baths. Morning, night, doesn't matter, I am taking a bath unless the tub won't hold water or there isn't a tub in the bathroom. I never questioned my love of baths until I got older, when "other people" told me all these reasons why I should not take baths and instead take showers. Their arguments were often something like this "Who has the time?" "You're sitting in a vat of your filth?" "You're wasting water!" I am sure you have a few you could add to the list.

Various doctors agree baths are, without a doubt, the more relaxing choice. Dermatologist Doris Day, MD, says it can be great for your skin in the long run. "You can add ingredients into the bathwater to help treat the skin, which doesn't work in the shower," she says. "If you have aches and pains, you can add Epsom salt. If you have eczema, dry, irritated skin, or a sunburn, you can add oatmeal, whole milk, and honey." Dermatologist Whitney Bowe, MD, adds that baths can lower cortisone levels, which in turn helps delay premature aging and reduce acne. She recommends using the soak-and-smear technique (soak for 10 minutes, then pat on moisturizer or oil as soon as you step out). Baths help lower cortisol levels in the body. Cortisol is a stress hormone that can increase acne and induce premature aging. Dr. Bowe also recommends avoiding any products that foam because they usually contain detergents, which strip the skin of natural, good-for-you oils. Soaking with any of these detergents in the water for too long will dry out your skin. Another aspect of baths is the temperature. If your bath is too hot, you're at risk of causing dryness because of the heat.

There's nothing more relaxing than a long, soak in the tub, but let me share with you a few more reasons why baths could be right for you and some of the benefits of wonderful tub time.

Heat can provide excellent relief for our inflamed or sore muscles. Medical News Today explains, applying heat can help your muscles relax. In a bath, you can fully submerge yourself in warm water, which relieves the muscles throughout your body. Adding Epsom salt can help reduce the aches and pains as well.

Please, put aside your worries about baths being unhygienic. Dr. Day says sitting in bathwater is far from filthy. "The dirt tends to settle away from the skin and body. It gets diluted in the entirety of the bathwater" Finally if you are worried about the water, make sure to add Epsom salt and baking soda in the water before you get in which will aid in keeping the water clean and safe. I understand a lot of people feel that baths are somehow "dirtier" than showers since the water isn't draining, but this isn't true. But if you are covered in yuck and muck wash off with your garden hose before going into your home. If you are inside already, take a shower before attempting a bath.

Try a little experiment that may open your eyes a bit. In some way make both of your hands as messy as possible. Possibly go outside and dig in your flowerbed, change the oil in your car, I am sure you can think of a messy activity. After your hands are nice and dirty wash one hand off with soap and water under the faucet. Place the other hand in a bowl of warm water with baking soda and Epsom salt and soak for 5 minutes. Those of you that think showers are so much cleaner will be surprised to see how the hand soaked in Epson salt come out. Salt is a natural disinfectant also. Unless you are bathing after someone else, you are not using dirty water or sitting in your "waste," but if you are uncomfortable, you can rinse off in the shower before and after you bathe. Or if you still question me take one of the strips that test pool water and check your bath water after you have bathed.

Now let's move on to health benefits of taking a nice warm bath. Scientists now say that taking a hot bath burns a ton of calories! No matter how active you are, taking a hot bath should be a part of your fitness routine. Did you know, climbing in the tub and taking a relaxing bath burns as many calories as a half-hour of gentle exercise? Even more surprising, taking a hot bath had a profound effect on blood sugar levels. Scientists in the U.K. and the U.S. recently discovered that taking a warm bath can reduce your blood sugar levels. These studies were with participants who had their peak glucose (blood sugar) levels monitored. After taking a hot bath, participants' glucose levels were 10% lower than they were after exercise. The researcher leading the study, Dr. Steve Faulkner, believes that being submerged in the heat of a hot bath causes the body to release heat shock proteins, which burn up the glucose at an unusually high rate of speed. Obviously, a nice soak in the tub should not replace exercise and healthy eating, but it can be a great addition! If you have blood sugar issues, talk to your doctor about taking a bath after you work out for a "one-two-punch."

According to TubYoga, increasing your body temperature can improve circulation, calm your nervous system, detoxify your body, and release endorphins. These endorphins make you feel good and can get rid of the stress that builds up throughout the day. To make it even more relaxing, light a scented candle, add some baking soda, Epsom salt and drip essential oils into the bath for some at-home aromatherapy.

Some excellent essential oils for relieving stress are jasmine, rose, lavender, clary sage (only a tiny amount because too much can cause a headache), sandalwood, geranium (pregnant and nursing women should not use this oil), Epsom Salt and ylang-ylang.

Eucalyptus, spearmint and peppermint are three excellent essential oils to ease congestion and help people breathe a little easier.

I must admit with my age number climbing, so does my blood pressure. Great news baths have been proven to lower blood pressure, which decreases stress on the heart and the cardiovascular system. Finally, if you ask anyone that knows me, they will tell you I am a firm believer that every woman should take every bath with Epsom salt at a minimum of twice a week and soak for at least ten minutes. "Women need magnesium to help combat common health conditions like premenstrual syndrome (PMS), hormonal migraines, anxiety, and depression," says the author of Super Woman RX Dr. Tasneem Bhatia ("Dr. Taz").

There are a lot of myths "floating around" about why baths aren't as good for you like showers, but I hope I have been able to dispel some of them. If you're washing off from a typical day, a bath will get you just as clean as a shower. Plus, the steam from a bath can open up your pores and release the dirt. Be a little creative and use essential oils you prefer and make your very own unique feel-better bath or whatever you decide to name it. Baths may take a bit longer, but I believe I am worth those few extra minutes just for me!

Now, where did you put your rubber ducky and glass of wine?

Feel-Better Bath

This bath is one of my favorites for relieving stress:

Ingredients

     10 drops of Jasmine Oil

6 drops of Lavender Oil

6 drops of Sandalwood Oil

1 quart of Distilled Water

6 ounces of liquid Castile Soap (this is an Olive Oil-based soap)

6 ounces of liquid Glycerin

Directions

Mix the water, soap, and glycerin then stir, while adding your essential oils to the mixture. Making sure to store in a dark glass airtight container. Add 1/4 cup of your essential oil mixture along with 1/2 cup baking soda and 1 cup Epsom salt (double ingredients for large tubs) under running water while the bath is filling. Relax and soak for twenty minutes without distractions. Turn off the telephone and turn on some soothing music.

Salt and Herb Bath

All spas, I have been to have a "Salt Glow." The salt helps to exfoliate the top layer of skin, thus removing the dead stuff and leaving a subtle "glow." You can DIY this very quickly.

Ingredients:

Sea Salt

Almond Oil

Eucalyptus or Peppermint Essential Oil.

Alternatively, you can use fresh Lavender or Rosemary herbs.

Directions:

Fill your bathtub with warm water. Add sea salt, few drops of almond oil. After that, you may add a few drops of eucalyptus or peppermint essential oil or if you have fresh rosemary and lavender plants even better. Sit back, relax, and soak away all the day's stress. Whenever you are using oil in your bathtub or shower, remember to please be careful about exiting. Most likely, all surfaces that have come in contact with the oil will have become very slippery.

Fabulous and Fizzy Bombshell

Add a little ball of fizz that dissolves in hot water while adding a slight scent and moisture to your bath. These bath bombs are my kind of bombs, and very easy to make at home.

Ingredients

1/2 cup Cornstarch

1/2 cup Ground Epsom Salt to a fine powder

3/4 cup Baking Soda

1/2 cup Citric Acid

3/4 tablespoon Water

Essential Oil (of your choice)

4 tablespoons Monoi Oil

Your choice Food Coloring (Optional)

Directions:

Mix your dry ingredients and the wet in a separate bowl.

Combine the two bowls quickly. Whisk and blend until you get a mix the consistency of wet sand. You'll also need something to shape the bath bombs. I used my cookie scoop to mold bath bombs. Pack the mixture in really tight and turn upside down on a cookie sheet. If you get one that doesn't come out in one piece, don't stress. Just plop it back into the bowl and re-shape it. Let your bath bombs dry overnight then wrap them in cellophane or place in an airtight storage container.

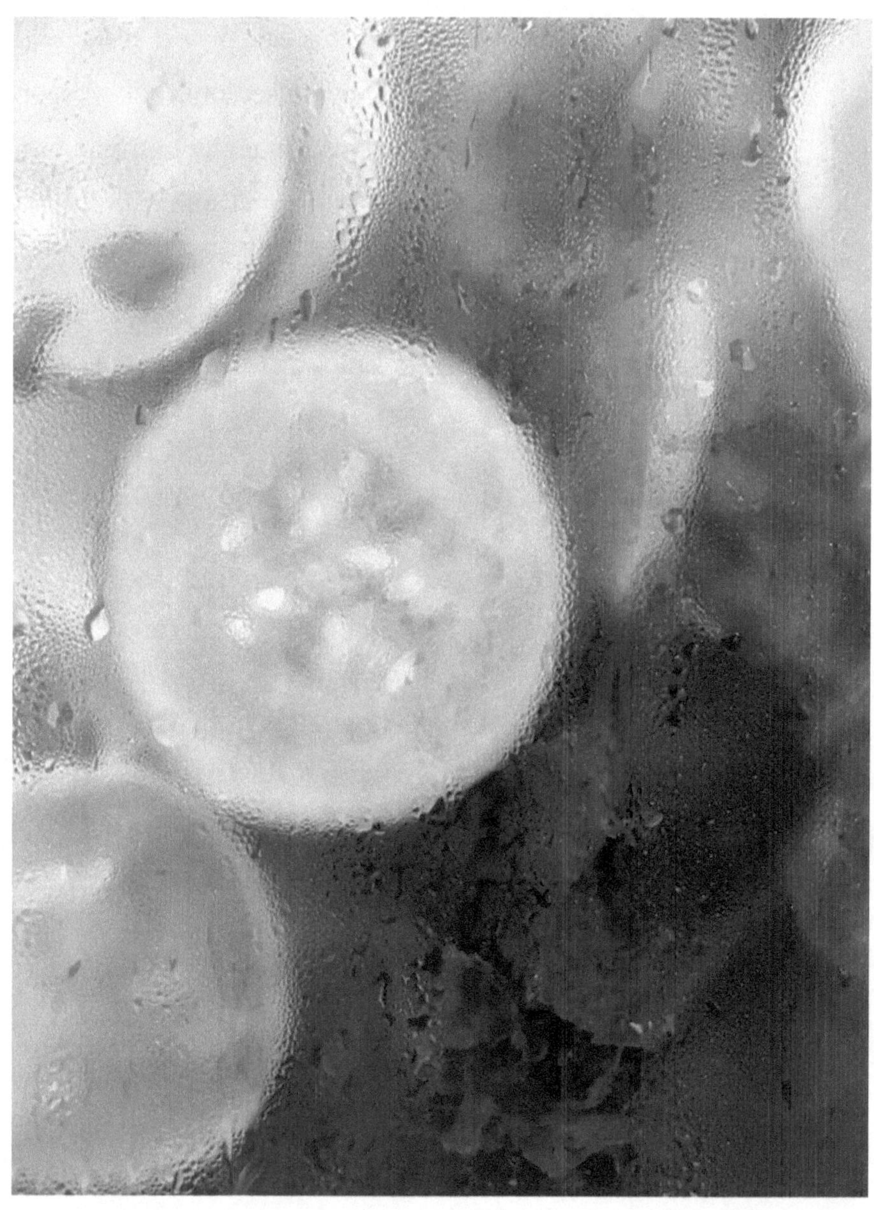

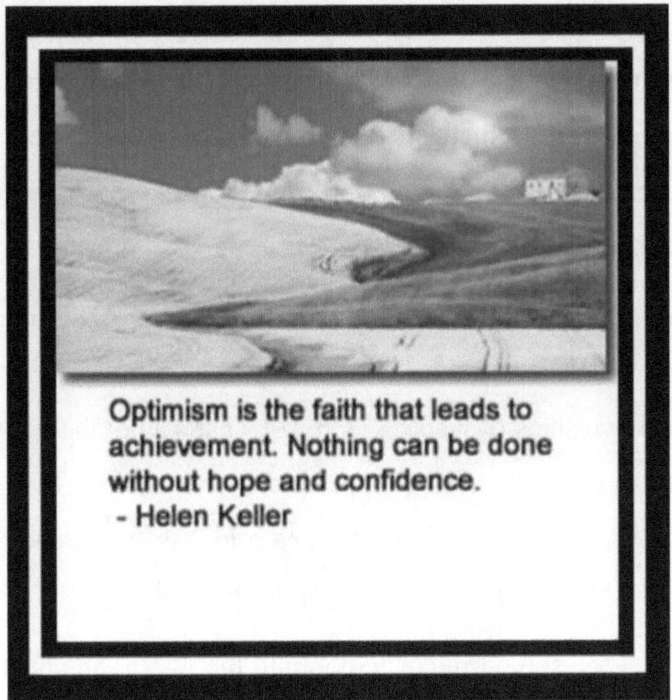

Chapter 4

Beauty Starts Inside

[This chapter is excerpted from the Divorced and Scared NO More series book 2 Practical Advice for the Newly Divorced   by Tasher]

Advantages of Drinking Water

You may be wondering why I am talking about drinking water in a divorce self-help book. It's because drinking water is one of the simplest things you can do that will help you feel tremendously better. Since most of our body mass is water, drinking eight glasses of water a day keeps us hydrated. (This needs to be adjusted depending on what type of climate you live in and how much you weigh). Remember, the body can only absorb four ounces of water every ten minutes, so don't try to drink your daily dose of water too quickly.

For those of you who complain that drinking water is boring: Boil it and brew strong tea, adding two tablespoons of honey, a splash of lemon and two shots of whiskey. Oh, no! That's a hot toddy, which is a tasty adult beverage during those cold winter nights. This yummy elixir is also known for helping get over a cold. You could also try some of these ideas to help make drinking water fun:

- Squeeze some lime or lemon into the water. The pectin fiber in lemons helps to fight hunger and assist in weight loss. Lemons and limes are packed full of vitamins and minerals, which will help with digestion and provide your body with an energy boost. The scent of lemons has a calming effect on your nervous system, which can help reduce anxiety and depression.
- Drink herbal and green teas without caffeine. They are good hot or cold and are available in a variety of flavors. Keep a pitcher of tea in the refrigerator, so it is ready when you are.
- In the morning, drink a glass of warm water with the juice of one lemon on an empty stomach to assist with detoxifying the liver and aid in weight loss.
- Invest in a water purifier and attach it to your kitchen tap or

get one of the pitcher types. Water filters can improve the taste of water tremendously.

Infused Water

Start your day by adding a generous amount of fresh mint leaves, strawberry, apple, lemon or lime to a pitcher of water. Now here is the problematic part: let the water sit for at least thirty minutes before drinking. You may find it easier to make this water as soon as you wake, so by the time you are done getting ready, it has had time to infuse. Keep a pitcher of your "fruit water" in the refrigerator, so you will always have the great-tasting water available.

Next is a list of things you can add to your water and what benefits they have.

- *Green Tea, Mint, and Lime:* fat burning, digestion, prevent headaches, helps with congestion and freshens breath
- *Strawberries and Kiwi:* cardiovascular health, immune system protection, blood sugar regulation, and digestion
- *Cucumber, Lime, and Lemon:* water weight management, bloating, appetite control, hydration, and digestion
- *Lemon, Lime, and Orange:* provides vitamin C, immune defense, digestion, heartburn (drink this type at room temperature for full benefit)

Herbal waters should be lightly flavored; you will only need a small number of herbs. They should gently infuse the water. Please show some restraint unless you are like me, a full-flavored gal. Some recipes call for steeping herbs in boiling water, which can change the flavor of the herbs, so try a little before you make a big batch.

You can add more water using the same fruit or herb base but discard after twenty-four hours. Now that you have a list of ingredients go out and create your special water. Be creative with herbs and tasty add-ins. Below are some of my favorite combinations to get you started.

Mint, Chocolate Mint or Apple Mint Herbal Water

Ingredients

>   Rinsed fresh Mint or Apple Mint
>   5 drops Double Chocolate Flavor Concentrate

Directions

>   Fill any travel cup or sports bottle with water, adding a few sprigs of mint or apple mint. Depending on how intense you want the flavor, make sure to slightly bruise some of the leaves, which will release the mint or apple mint oils into the water. A quick way to make chocolate mint water (one of our family favorites) is to add the double chocolate flavor concentrate. Refrigerate for a couple of hours before drinking.

Hibiscus tea is delicious, and it is reported to have many health benefits. Personally, it helps me with my blood pressure. Research has shown hibiscus can help you reduce your blood pressure, lose weight, and reduce bad cholesterol. Did you know hibiscus contains an enzyme inhibitor that blocks the amount of sugar absorbed by the body? Less sugar consumed means fewer pounds. Hibiscus also makes it more difficult for LDL cholesterol to bind to artery walls, resulting in reduced blockages. That's how it helps blood pressure and cholesterol. But since this section is about the infused water, not tea, here is a great recipe.

Hibiscus Star Fruit Orange Water

Ingredients

80 oz Water

2 teaspoons loose Hibiscus Tea (or two bags)

4 Orange slices

5 slices cored Star Fruit

Directions

Combine all ingredients in your pitcher. Chill for 4 to 12 hours. Not only do you have a great tasting beverage, but it is healthy to boot.

Some other delicious combinations for herbal infused water are listed below. Usually, I bruise herbs except for thyme. Merely bruise the herbs in your hand or stick them in a bag and whack it a couple of times with a wooden spoon to provide the right amount of bruising.

- Thinly sliced unpeeled cucumbers, lemons, spearmint and rosemary
- Lemongrass and lavender
- Lemon verbena, lemon peel, and thyme
- Lemongrass and mint

- Citrus peel, pineapple, and mint
- Strawberries and basil
- Cucumber and basil
- Thinly sliced oranges and sage

Passionflower Tea and Stress Relief

Tea has been around for thousands of years. Historically it has been used for medicine and relaxation. This tea is a refreshing addition to your diet and exercise regimen with stress-relieving benefits. Passionflower contains chrysin, and that is what provides anti-anxiety benefits. In 2011, researchers wrote in a journal called European Neuropsychopharmacology that "a number of human trials have evinced the anxiolytic or anti-anxiety, effects of passionflower."

Ingredients

1 tablespoon of the Dried Herbs
1 cup of Boiling Water
1 tablespoon of Honey (optional)

Directions

Add herbs to water, steep for 10 minutes, strain. If desired, add 1 tablespoon of Honey. Drink the tea near bedtime to assist with sleep.

Note: Please consult your healthcare professional before using passionflower tea. Pregnant or lactating women and children under the age of six should not use

passionflower because there are no studies of its effects on these groups of people. All recipes and suggestions within this book are merely suggestions. Nothing within this book should be used without the approval or as a substitute for whatever your medical professional recommends.

Frozen Fruit

As I have grown older, it has become harder and harder to avoid gaining weight. I was always known as the girl with a hollow leg because I could eat anything I wanted and not gain weight. But now I look at something, and the pounds come on. I have a bit of a sweet tooth and love dessert; ice cream is my favorite after-dinner treat. Deciding to cut calories first, I reached for frozen yogurt or sherbet. Then I found out that the calorie count per cup is 140 for frozen yogurt and 260 for sherbet. Frozen fruit is only 120 for a cup.

When bananas get a little too ripe, I peel the skin off, slice the bananas, and place them on a wax paper-lined cookie sheet in a single layer. Then I pop them in the freezer. Once they are frozen, I put them in a freezer-safe Ziploc type bag. It's the same process for other fruit. Make sure to clean and remove all stems before freezing.

I have a Yonana machine to make a soft-serve treat, but a good food processor can do the trick. I will warn you the Yonana machine is quite loud, and the frozen treat does not taste quite like ice cream, though it is delicious.

Another quick idea to satisfy your craving for sweets is to wash and freeze grapes or blueberries, making sure to eat them frozen.

Zesty Lemon Sorbet

If you've read my book series, *Divorced and Scared NO More,* this recipe will look familiar. It's a delicious treat that always reminds me that when life gives me lemons, I should make Zesty Lemon Sorbet!

Ingredients

> 1/2 cup Honey
>
> 3/4 cup Carbonated Mineral Water
>
> 3/4 cup fresh Lemon Juice
>
> 1 teaspoon Lemon Zest
>
> 4 shots low-calorie Lemon-flavored Vodka
>
> A drizzle of Lemon Liqueur to taste

Directions

> Mix honey, water, lemon juice, zest, and vodka. Pour into a shallow container and place in the freezer, fluffing with a fork occasionally until it is semi-frozen. Return to the freezer until frozen solid. Freeze overnight, in the morning remove it and let sit on the counter for a few minutes to thaw just a bit so you can break it up. Run it through a food processor or blender until smooth. Place sorbet in an airtight container and freeze until ready to serve.
>
> Serve as you would ice cream and drizzle with lemon liqueur

to taste.

Don't stop believing in yourself! Continue to eat healthily, drink your water, sing, and dream of blue skies over the rainbow.

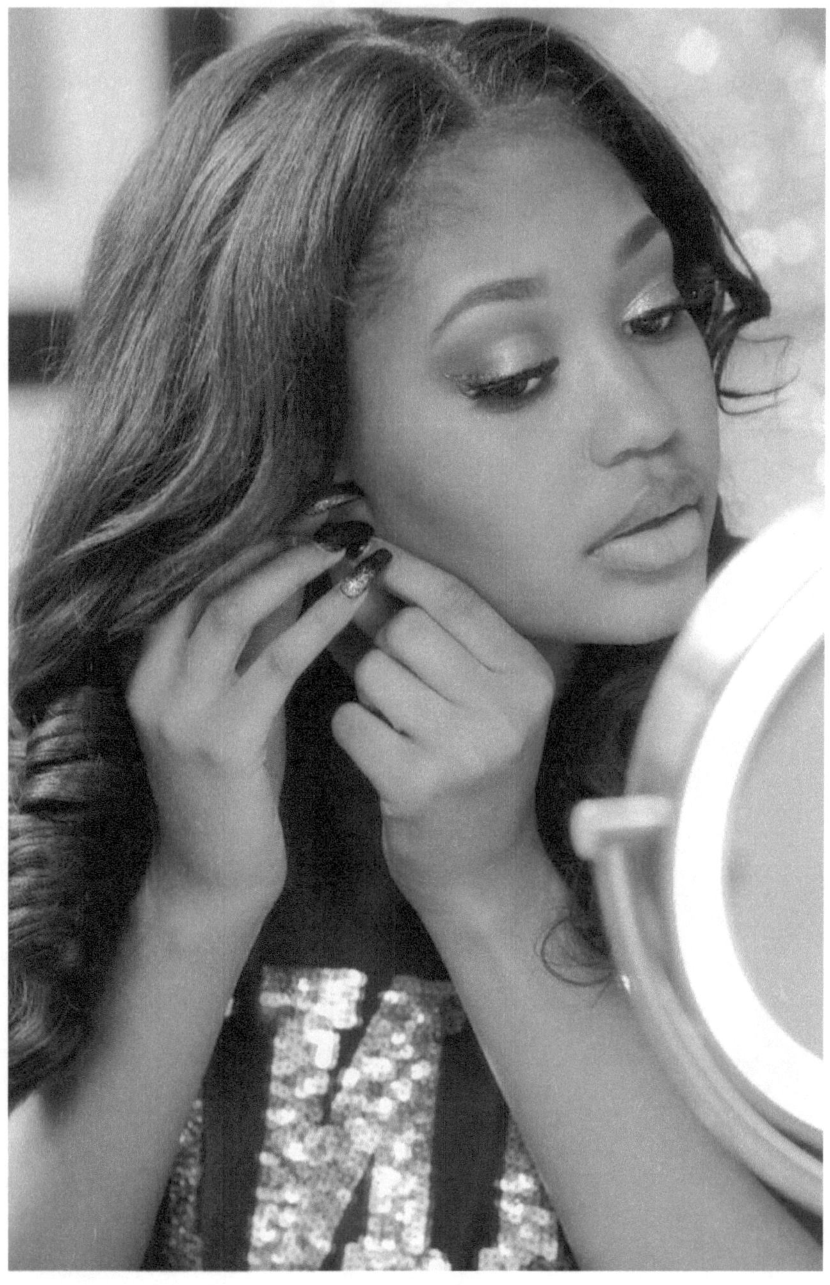

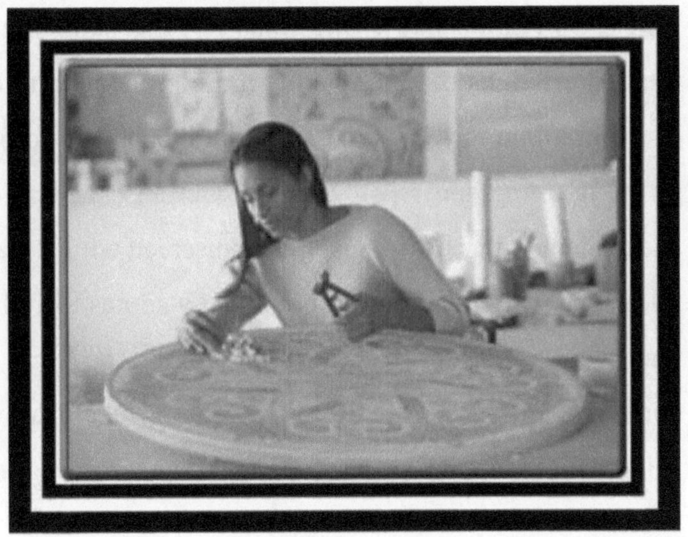

Chapter 5

Anti-Aging for Every Skin Tone

The pigment in your skin not only determines the type, texture, and color; it also plays a significant role in how your skin ages. You need to be aware of the differences and how it will affect your anti-aging skin routine. Everyone should have these basics in their skincare regimen: cleansing sun protection and additional products geared toward your skin type. Within each skin type, there also many skin tones. The darker the skin color is, the more melanin it has. The melanin will help as built-in sun protection, but everyone still needs sunscreen. Melanin absorbs some of the UV light, thus causing less damage to your skin.

Fair Skin (Caucasian): Unfortunately, this skin type shows the earliest signs of aging and is more prone to skin cancer. The biggest thing your skin type should focus on is protection in the morning and repair at night. Get an excellent quality antioxidant with a broad-spectrum sunscreen with at least SPF 30. For your foundation, find one that also has SPF then top that with a powder with SPF. At night, be sure to use corrective products with Retin-A, retinol, or alpha-hydroxy acids. This skin type is also prone to redness, rosacea, and age spots.

Olive Skin (Asian): This is the most sensitive skin type and is susceptible to sun damage, acne, and inflammation. Sun protection and very gentle products are essential. A soft, gentle multi-tasking product would be best for your skin type.

Olive Skin (Hispanic/Latina): Lighter Olive types are prone to sagging fine lines and pigmentation problems. Sun protection is a must. Retinol and Retin-A are outstanding night products for this skin type. Be very careful and start only using the product once or twice a week and build up based on how you react. Microdermabrasion or light chemical peels can help with uneven skin tone.

Darker Skin (South Asians/Middle Eastern): This skin tone seems to wrinkle less but are very prone to pigmentation problems and having dark patches. Sunscreen is a must for this skin type. Very often this skin tone will lose volume in their upper cheeks, which creates a hollow under eye appearance and makes the dark circles more noticeable. Dermatologists have many types of fillers they can suggest for assisting with these problems.

Very Dark Skin (African-American): On the plus side, you don't show aging signs as quickly as Caucasians. The negative side you're more prone to skin issues like scars raising, hyperpigmentation, and ingrown hairs. Moisturizers are essential for you but do not use moisturizers with oil. The best way to put on moisturizer is right after you get out of the shower while your skin is still a little wet. Even though you have a high melanin content in your skin sunscreen will always protect you and benefit your skin's overall appearance. Don't be fooled by the old wives' tale that because of your skin color, you cannot get a sunburn. That is a false statement. ANYONE exposed long enough will get a sunburn. Plus, there are so many benefits to using sunscreen it should be a must for everyone arsenal to fight the war and hold back the hands of time!

Congratulations you just completed your crash course on the differences in skin types. Hopefully, you can begin to create your regimen for skincare that will help you keep your fresh, youthful look.

Shake up That Makeup!

After 40, it is time to rethink how you do your make up! Just changing a few little things with a trick or two can help make those years a little less noticeable. So, take a few minutes and shake up that makeup!

Here are some tips for updating your look:

- **Go One Darker** - Get foundation one shade darker. Many people go one shade lighter, and that works well for younger people, but as we age, our skin is not as even of a tone. Those little spots start showing up. A lighter color does not blend as well, but one shade darker will do the trick. Not only will it give you a younger look, but it also adds a warm glow to your skin.

- **Use Bronzer** - Bring a little life and lift to your face by making sure you bring out the bones of your face. Apply the bronzer right on your facial bones, start at two fingers from the nose and go up with your check bone then down on your jaw bone.

- **Blush It Up** - Place your blush higher on the cheekbone and follow the cheekbone all the way up to your temple. Applying blush in this manner can give the illusion of lift.

- **For Lips, less is More** - Use a light-colored lipstick with no blue undertones. A product I will not go without is Sally Hanson Lip Inflation. It does work to plump up your lips. Don't be afraid to use a bright red during the holiday, but this should be saved for special occasions. The everyday look should be lighter and simpler.

- **Lift Your Eyes** - When applying any shadow or eyeliner, always end with an upward motion, this will create the illusion of a lift. If your eyebrows are thinning, fill them in softly with an eyebrow pencil. I have had microblading done and would recommend it highly. As with anything permanent or semi-permanent, PLEASE do your homework and check the people doing the service out. Read their reviews and see photos of how their final work looks. You don't want a botched job and have to go elsewhere to get things fixed.

- **Powder Only in the Center** - Only powder the center of your face. When you do the other areas, it mattes down the whole face, plus using too much powder also magnifies the wrinkles.

Age-Fighting Foods to Look and Feel Younger

Your beauty and health will start on the inside and work its way out. Remember the old saying, "You are what you eat" Well, it is very accurate! If you are unhealthy, your appearance will mirror how you feel. You will not look glowing and youthful if your biological clock says you are 40, but due to inadequate healthcare, your internal body clock says 80. I like most would like to look less than my age and never look twice my age. Here are some diet tips that will help you look and feel younger.

- **Reduce your carbohydrates and sugar intake:** Most of us eat way too many carbs and sugar. Did you know elevated amounts of sugar can make change your blood markers as quickly as ten weeks? Abnormal levels of triglycerides increase your danger of having heart diseases and stroke. The benefits of a low carb and sugar diet may help prevent or improve dangerous health conditions.

- **Whole Grain Pasta:** Whole grain pasta has three times more antioxidants than other pasta. Whole grains reduce the risk of heart disease. To make sure you are getting what you are paying for the whole wheat should be listed as the first ingredient.

- **Coconut Water:** Coconuts are very high in antioxidants and are reported to help diabetes, heart disease, and the big one is high blood pressure.

- **Eggs:** Eggs have the antioxidant lutein which protects your eyes from macular degeneration and cataracts. Because the amount was low, people usually would go for spinach. Research has found the lutein in the yolk of the egg is absorbed better by the body than it is with spinach.

- **Canola Oil or Olive Oil:** Either of these is considered to be heart-healthy oils.

- **Canned Beans:** There are high levels of antioxidants in specific beans. The rule of thumb is the darker the vegetable is, the better it is for you.

- **Popcorn:** Popcorn has a cancer-fighting plant compound. Air-popped is the best way to have your popcorn.

- **Yogurt:** Eating 1 cup of low-fat plain yogurt will provide at least 25 percent of the daily value for riboflavin (a B vitamin). Did you know why Greek yogurt is different? The extra whey has been strained out of the yogurt, which makes it a bit thicker, creamier, and tangy. Usually plain has less sugar and more protein than flavored yogurt. Yogurt delivers twice the bone-strengthening mineral calcium.

If you notice this list is full of excellent food, you probably have in your kitchen right now. Hopefully, you can see that you can eat healthy food that also tastes good.

Wrinkle Reducer Recipes

I hate to be the one to tell you if you're looking for a face-lift in a bottle, you probably won't find it! The benefits of these products are usually only modest at best. The effectiveness of anti-wrinkle creams mostly depends on the active ingredient or ingredients. Here are some common ingredients that can help achieve some improvement in the appearance of wrinkles. **Retinol** is a vitamin A compound. It is an antioxidant used in many nonprescription wrinkle creams. **Vitamin C.** is another potent antioxidant; vitamin C may help protect skin from sun damage. **Alpha hydroxy acids, beta hydroxy acids (salicylic acid), and polyhydroxy acids** are all excellent exfoliants. **Coenzyme Q10** has shown promise in various studies to help reduce fine wrinkles around the eyes and protect the skin from sun damage.

Peptides have been used in products for wound healing, stretch marks, and now wrinkles. **Green, black, and oolong tea extracts** contain compounds with antioxidant and anti-inflammatory properties. In addition to its antioxidant properties, **Grape seed extract** also has anti-inflammatory properties and promotes wound healing. Finally, a very potent antioxidant is **Niacinamide**, which is related to vitamin B-3 (niacin). It helps reduce water loss in the skin and may improve skin elasticity.

Below you will find what many members of the DASNM (Divorced and Scared NO More) community have called their must-haves. Many people experiment by taking the items mentioned above and mixing them with the things mentioned below. DIY beauty care is supposed to be a fun way for you to create your very own, amazing, rejuvenating products, created especially for you by you. It is our grown-up version of when we were kids playing with our science kit or easy bake oven.

- *Banana* - Mash banana and spread all over your face and leave for 10 minutes. Rinse with warm water.

- *Green Grapes* - All you do is squash grapes and gently apply on your face and neck. Leave on for 10 minutes rinse with warm water.

- *Use Vitamin E oil* – Wash your face then break open a vitamin E oil capsule and dab it all over your face with a fingertip where the lines are, making sure to get around the eyes. Follow the same process with either Jojoba or

Frankincense oil. For around your eye area mix Vitamin E oil with **Aloe Vera gel**.

- ***Foods to Eat*** - Omega-3 Fatty Acids are found in salmon, halibut, sardines, albacore, trout, herring, walnut, flaxseed oil, and canola oil. Other foods that contain omega-3-fatty acids include shrimp, clams, light chunk tuna, catfish, cod, and spinach. Omega-6 fatty acids are found in corn, safflower, sunflower, soybean and cottonseed oil.

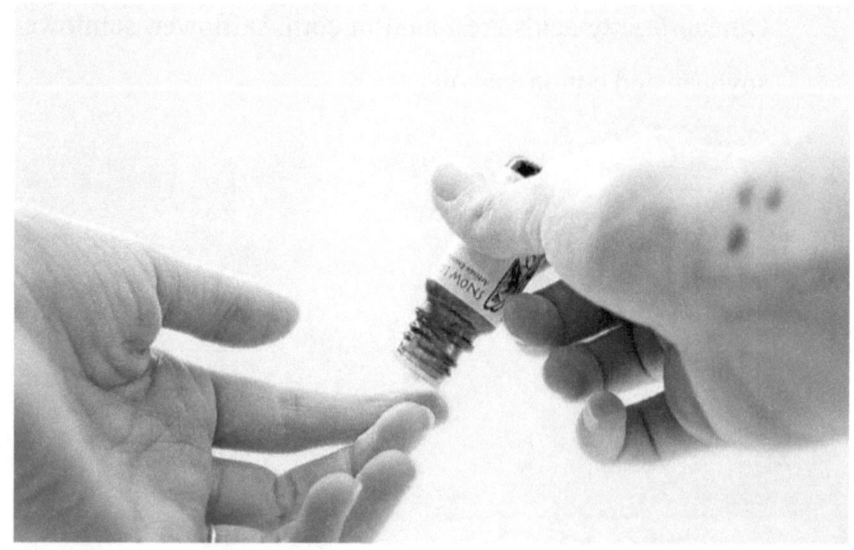

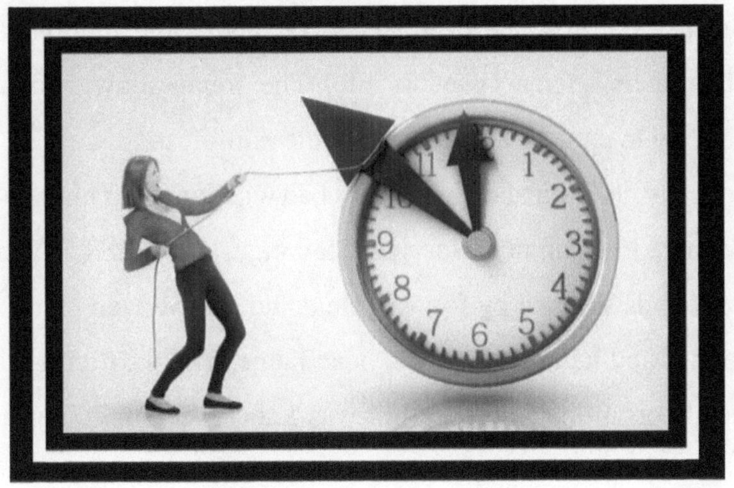

Chapter 6

Could Monoi Oil Be Your Next Best Beauty Secret?

I had never heard of Monoi oil until I moved to the Philippine Islands. My ex-husband was one of the pilots that helped FedEx start their worldwide operation. For him to do his job, keep the family together plus give our children an experience of a lifetime, we packed up the family (pets included) and moved to Subic Bay. Anyone that knows me will tell you I make friends quickly from all walks of life. Including the people that lived in the rainforest behind our home. Negritos worked as instructors in the Jungle Warfare School at Subic Bay naval base until it closed in November 1992. Negritos still guide tourists through the 32,000-acre jungle, one of the last areas of tropical rainforest on Luzon Island. Working as guides enable the Negritos, the original inhabitants of the Philippines, to maintain their ancient way of life. The tours allow visitors an opportunity to explore and appreciate the rainforest.

One-day my children and I had a very bad windburn. On his way back from Jungle Environment Survival Training Camp (JEST, one of my jungle friends stopped by to visit. He could see we were not feeling well at all, and he quickly left to head home. The next thing I knew my neighbors from down the hill was knocking at my door again. This time he was handing me a jar of a wonderful elixir his wife had sent for us. Sometimes the Negritos make things out of stuff I would rather NOT know what was in it. I was in pain but seeing my children hurting so badly I was willing to try anything to help all of us feel better. I decided not to ask but instead say thank you and give it a try. I was so shocked the next morning when I got out of bed, and there was NO pain. I realized I had slept all night, and the kids also did! Now, I had to know what this grand elixir was that helped everyone in my family feel better practically overnight and who cares what the ingredients are! The next time I saw my friend, I asked if I could come down to the village with him to see his wife. When I arrived at camp my friend's wife told me about Monoi (pronounced Mah-noy) oil. It is very simple to make by soaking Rosal' flowers (the U.S. closest flower is a Gardenia) and coconut oil.

Like many things in the Philippine Islands, the roots for this oil can be traced elsewhere. The date when monoi was first created is unknown; however, its origins can be traced back over 2000 years to the Maohi people, the indigenous Polynesians. Monoï is widely used among French Polynesians as a skin and hair softener. The Maohi tribe used this oil from birth till death for medical, cosmetic, and religious reasons. Uses for Monoi oil included protecting the skin from harsh winds, saltwater and prevent dehydration of the skin in hot weather. After a death, the tribe embalmed the bodies with the oil to assist in the journey to the afterlife. The Priests also use it in religious rituals anointing objects and purifying offerings.

Negritos DIY Monoi Oil

Directions:

1. Collect enough Gardenia flowers to fill a clean, sterilized, and cooled mason jar. Take all the petals off and put them in the jar one at a time. Do not pack the flower petals in too tight but make sure to fill the jar with the loose petals.

2. Fill the jar with Coconut Oil. Put the lid on the jar, so no liquid leaks out but making sure not to overtighten.

3. Shake once or more a day for a month, making sure the oil jar gets at least 4 hours a day in sunlight. Then strain the petals from the Mason jar making sure to squeeze out each little drop of your oil. At this point to have a little bit of extra fun pretend you are Gollum from the Hobbit. As you stoke and squeeze your oil, calling it "my precious…". Go ahead, have fun. One of my friends told

me, "the more fun I have making it, the more potent it will be."

4.   Pour the strained oil, into a clean sterilized dark blue or brown jar and store in a cool dark place.

Using the monoi oil scrubs daily can seriously improve your skin; it also happens to be one of the easiest most natural products to make! My favorite is to make a simple scrub. Add monoi oil with Epsom salt and scrub my body then carefully rinse off in the shower, followed by tapping my body dry with the towel. The reason I tap dry is to keep as much monoi oil on my skin as possible. My over 50-year-old skin needs it way more than the towel does.

In the Buff Scrubs

Scrubs are a great way to use your monoi oil. The recipes below will help you get started on your own DIY body scrub collection. Remember that substitutions are possible, so mix and match to make it your own.

Beauty Bliss Facial Scrub

Ingredients:

2 drops of Almond Essential Oil

2 drops Monoi Oil

1 cup of Oatmeal

Directions:

Mix and store in a dark glass airtight container. When using this scrub, wet your hands and apply the paste on your face in a circular motion to peel away the dead skins. Rinse with water.

Healing Wings Hand and Foot Scrub

Ingredients:

1 cup Epsom Salt

1 tablespoon Petroleum Jelly

1/4 cup Monoi Oil

Crushed Orange or Lemon Peel, depending on your preferences.

Directions:

Mix well in a bowl. Taking small handfuls, rub into your hands and feet to remove the top layer of dead cells. Do this in a basin, sink or footbath because it can get a little messy. Rinse off and pat to dry your skin dry with the towel.

Scrubalicious Shower Scrub

Ingredients:

1 cup Epsom Salt

1/4 cup Monoi Oil

5 capsules of Vitamin E

5 capsules of Vitamin A

Lavender Oil or dried Lavender optional

Directions:

Mix Epsom Salt and Monoi Oil

Squeeze the oils from the vitamin capsules into the mixture

If desired, add a few drops of Lavender oil or dried lavender flowers.

Mix well in a bowl. Taking small handfuls, rub the scrub all over your body gently to remove the top layer of dead cells right before you get out of the shower. Then rinse off the scrub off with warm water.

Be very careful with any products with oil because it can make the floor very slippery. So, to avoid a fall, it is best to do this treatment in a shower equipped with proper anti-slip protection. After you get out of the shower pat to dry your skin, then rub into your skin any residual lotion. Your skin will feel silky smooth, show fewer wrinkles, and the creepy skin will be much less noticeable.

Mocha Scrub

Ingredients:

1/2 cup Monoi Oil

2/3 cup Coffee Grounds

1/3 cup Epsom Salt

5 drops Essential Oil of your choice

Directions:

Mix well together. Scrub a generous amount in a circular motion making sure to spend more time on the roughest patches of skin. Thoroughly rinse your skin to remove all leftover granules.

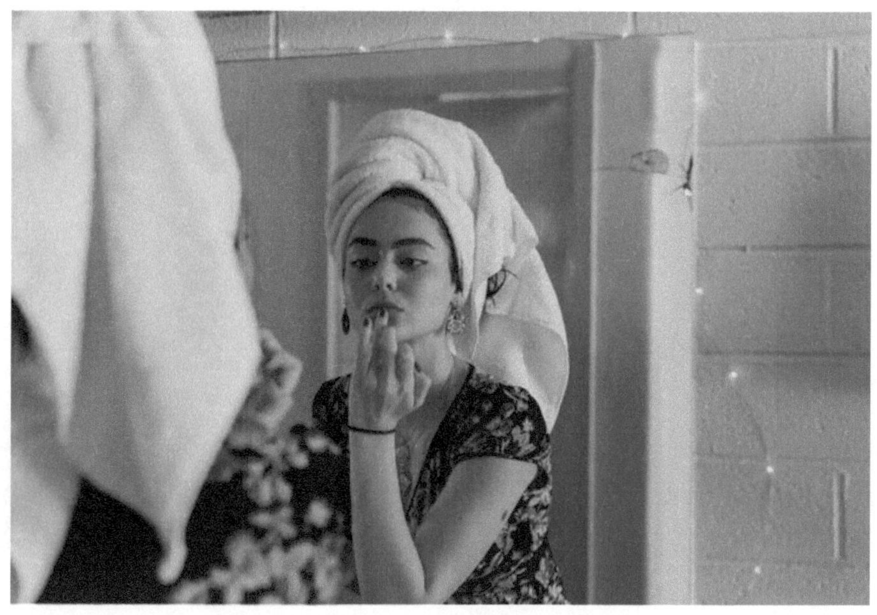

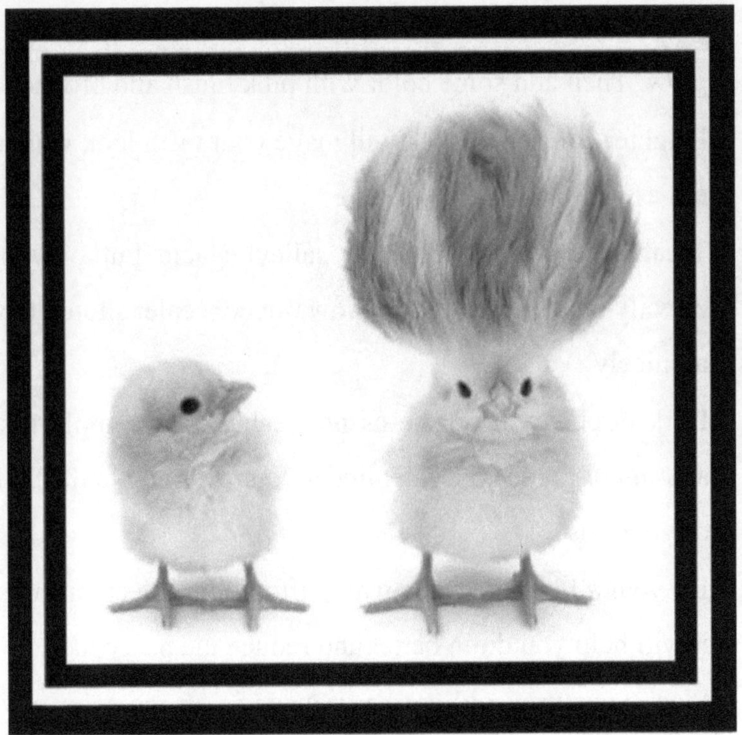

Chapter 7

Beauty Fixes

Just like bad hair days, we all have a terrible beauty day here and there. By using some of these tips and tricks, you can look great even if you don't feel great! Salon and spa owners in the Houston area shared a few tips and tricks they share with their customers.

- When your skin starts looking dull, exfoliate to get a beautiful glow. Then add some color with pink blush and bronzer.

- Brighter colored lipstick will make your teeth look whiter and not as yellow.

- Treat acne with glycolic or salicylic acid but only put it directly on the pimple. A yellow tint concealer should cover it up nicely.

- Dark circles will not be as noticeable if you apply a small amount of green concealer under your eyes and to the hollows of your nose.

- Do your allergies have you all puffy? If you sleep propped up, it will help you drain better and reduce the puffy face.

- Place your used old coffee grounds in an ice-cube tray and freeze. When your face is a bit puffy pull a cube out of the freezer and place it on your closed eye to remove the puffiness. The caffeine will get the circulation going while the coolness will reduce the puffy face problem.

Body Refreshers

The DASNM community also wanted to share their DIY Body refreshers that can give a little extra boost at the tip of your fingers when needed. The following recipes for body refreshers are easy to make and even easier to use. These body refreshers can be stored in small spray containers so you can have freshness on the go.

Body Spray

Ingredients:

> 2 cups White Vinegar
>
> 1/4 cup Honey
>
> 1 teaspoon Sage
>
> 1/4 teaspoon Vitamin C Powder

Directions

> Combine all ingredients in a sterilized glass mason. For 1-week, store and shake well every day. After one week, strain and pour into a spray bottle.

Hair Refresher and Curls Reviver

You will need a small Spray Bottle

1 to 2 Tbsp. Extra Virgin Coconut Oil

Fill 1/4 of the bottle with Aloe Juice

Fill remainder of the bottle with Distilled Water, about one inch of space at the top

Pour mixture into a microwave-safe container till microwave mixture until it is warm (only about 20 or 30 seconds)

Add 1 tsp of Epsom Salt and stir until dissolved

Pour back into the spray bottle and shake well to mix before each use. Depending on which has the best result for your hair type use one of these methods either after shampoo and rinse with water or spray on dry hair in the morning, scrunch hair and let hair air dry.

Green Tea Face Mist

Make Green Tea and let the bag sit in boiled water for 20 minutes. Add the tea to a spray bottle then add, Vitamin C powder and drop of Vitamin E oil. Mix well. Keep in the fridge before use. Mist your face when you want to cool down from the summer heat or just refreshed and relaxed. The antioxidants in this mix will make your skin jump with joy!

Foot Deodorizer

Mix 1 tsp. of Baking Soda and 2-3 drops of Peppermint Essential Oil Break apart the clumps then lightly dust your feet with the powder.

Some Honey, Honey?

Raw honey is incredible for your skin thanks to its antibacterial properties and a hefty serving of skin-saving antioxidants.

- Acne: Honey is naturally antibacterial, so it's great for acne treatment and prevention.
- Aging: Full of antioxidants, honey is great to slow down the hands of time and that darn aging clock.
- Complexion boost: Honey will help create a new glow because it is incredibly moisturizing and soothing.
- Pores: Honey is clarifying because it opens up pores, making them easy to unclog.

Below you will find a few recipes for some great uses for honey. Remember these are just suggestions to get you started. Please experiment with the formulas till tailor make one that suits your specific needs.

DIY Honey Mask

As mentioned earlier, raw honey can help unclog pores while delivering moisture to dry skin.

In a circular motion, apply a thin layer of raw honey to the slightly dampened skin. Leave on for 30 minutes and then gently rinse it off with warm water.

HST (Honey Spot Treatment)

Are you suffering from a breakout? Mix one tablespoon of honey with three drops of tea tree oil and two drops of lavender oil. Swirl a small amount of honey mixture on a cotton swab and dab onto your blemish.

Honey Cleanser

Mix honey with coconut or jojoba oil till it is slippery enough to slide across your face. Add in a dash of cinnamon, turmeric or nutmeg then massage over your face, loosening up heavy makeup and moisturizing your skin at the same time.

DIY Honey Exfoliator

Exfoliate from head to toe once or twice a week with the following gentle scrub. Use two parts honey and one-part Arm & Hammer Baking Soda. Mix well and scrub away.

Honey Bath

Add two cups of honey as your bath is filling. Soak for 15 minutes and then add a cup of Arm & Hammer Baking Soda and one cup Epson salt for your final 15 minutes.

Rosemary Oil and Your Hair

Rosemary Essential Oil is my favorite essential oil. Saying it is versatile could be a little of an understatement. Rosemary is used for eliminating harmful bacteria, improve concentration, relieve stress, calming nerves, calm digestive issues, encouraging hair growth, and the list goes on. It is frequently used in lotions or oils to relieve aching muscles and through aromatherapy.

Greek scholars started using rosemary to enhance their memory skills when taking exams. For thousands of years, people also used Rosemary and Lavender for its strengthening ability. Mark Moss, Jenny Cook, Keith Wesnes, and Paul Duckett conducted a study regarding "How the Aromas of Rosemary and Lavender Essential Oils Differently Affect Cognition and Mood in Healthy Adults." The results of this study were published on the 7th of July 2009, highlighting this phenomenon

Recently, a few other uses for rosemary have become popular. When applied to the scalp rosemary essential oil is credited to help stimulate hair growth. Many people claim that it can be used to prevent and treat dandruff.

Rosemary oil is a natural remedy, but that doesn't mean it is safe for everyone or in any concentration. As with the other various DIY ideas you find in this book, there are several things people should remember before using any essential oil. Women who are pregnant or breastfeeding should not use rosemary oil unless a doctor advises them. People should also avoid getting rosemary oil in their eyes or mouths. Always keep all essential oils out of reach of children. There is also no evidence that rosemary oil works for childhood hair loss or that it is safe to use on child's scalp. Consult your healthcare provider before starting any other recommendations in this book on yourself or your child. Your healthcare provider will know what is best for you and your family. Something that may work for me could interfere with something you use, such as a medication.

Most people wash their hair too much and strip their scalp of their essential natural oils. Stop washing your hair every day. Use Rosemary shampoo and conditioner each time you wash your hair use. Just add 10-12 drops of rosemary oil in 1 ounce of shampoo or conditioner. If you use hair oil or want to encourage hair growth, the recipe below does a fantastic job.

Rosemary Hair Oil

- 8 drops Rosemary Essential Oil
- 6 drops Lavender Essential Oil
- 3 drops of Clary Sage Essential Oil
- 2 tsp Castor Oil
- 1 tsp Coconut Oil
- 1 tsp Almond Oil
- Oil from 1 Vitamin E Capsules

This oil is said to encourage hair growth not only on the scalp but also on other areas you want to grow hair such as your eyebrows or beard. Make it a habit to shake all oils before applying since essential oils tend to separate after sitting for even a few minutes. Often, they do not mix but rather layer in the container. As mentioned before essential oils are best stored in a cool dark place in a dark glass container. I prefer dark blue or brown glass bottles with a dropper or spray. In this instance, the dropper makes it easier to apply to the scalp.

Do you remember hanging upside down from the monkey bars or tree branches when you were a kid? A modified version of this childhood pastime that encourages hair growth is called inversion therapy, and it has worked for many people around the world.

Scientists have theorized that one of the main components for maintaining acceptable hair growth is proper scalp circulation, particularly the microcirculation surrounding the hair follicles. The inversion method or hanging upside down while rubbing your head is meant to increase the blood flow to the scalp. Doing so for a few minutes is supposed to cause your hair follicles to reach maximum capacity and stimulate growth.

Most people have reported treatment is much more effective when using three or four tablespoons of warm Rosemary Hair Oil.

Instead of heating in a microwave or on the stove, place the bottle of oil in a bowl of warm water. This way, the oil can heat slowly while not losing any of its potency or getting too hot. Think about the way we used to warm baby bottles. Let the oil sit in the water for a few minutes or until the oil bottle is warm to the touch. Be careful not to overheat the oil; you do not want to burn your scalp accidentally!

After the oil is warm, it is time to massage the oils into your scalp. Set a timer for at least four minutes and begin your scalp massage. Once you have finished rubbing in the Rosemary Hair oil into your scalp, it is time for the inversion part of this treatment. Find a comfortable position and tip your head upside down in a relaxing way. There are many ways you can achieve the upside-down position:

- Leaning over a sink or bathtub
- Sitting upside down in a chair with your feet hanging over the back
- Laying on an inversion table if you have one

The final step in the inversion therapy is to wash your hair and scalp using your homemade rosemary shampoo and conditioner (recipe above).

To best facilitate hair growth, you should perform the inversion method for hair growth for one week, once a day, every three weeks. On the two off-weeks give yourself a daily 4-minute dry scalp massage.

If you have a dry scalp, after doing the inversion and before washing your hair, you may want to leave the oil on your scalp for an hour or so. If you choose to leave the oil on a bit longer, please remove excess oil and cover your oily scalp with a plastic wrap or shower cap. To prevent the oil from ruining your furniture or clothing. Do not leave the treatment on your hair any longer than one hour because it can clog your pores and inhibit hair growth.

It is crucial not to do inversion oil therapy too frequently. Excessive use of oil also can clog your pores because you have too much oil, and it will deter hair growth. But you can use your homemade Rosemary Shampoo and Conditioner daily if desired. You should start seeing results after about four months of dedicated treatments.

Note: The recommendation is that you do NOT use the oil or do inversion therapy on children or if you are pregnant or nursing. Short periods of inversion are typically good for your health, avoid excessive lengths of time upside down.

DO NOT attempt the inversion method for hair growth if you:

- *Have low blood pressure*
- *Have high blood pressure*
- *Have a detached retina*

- *Have a spinal injury*
- *Have a hernia*
- *Have an ear infection*

Make sure to consult with your healthcare provider before making any of the recommendations in this book, including inversion therapy, part of you or your families' routine.

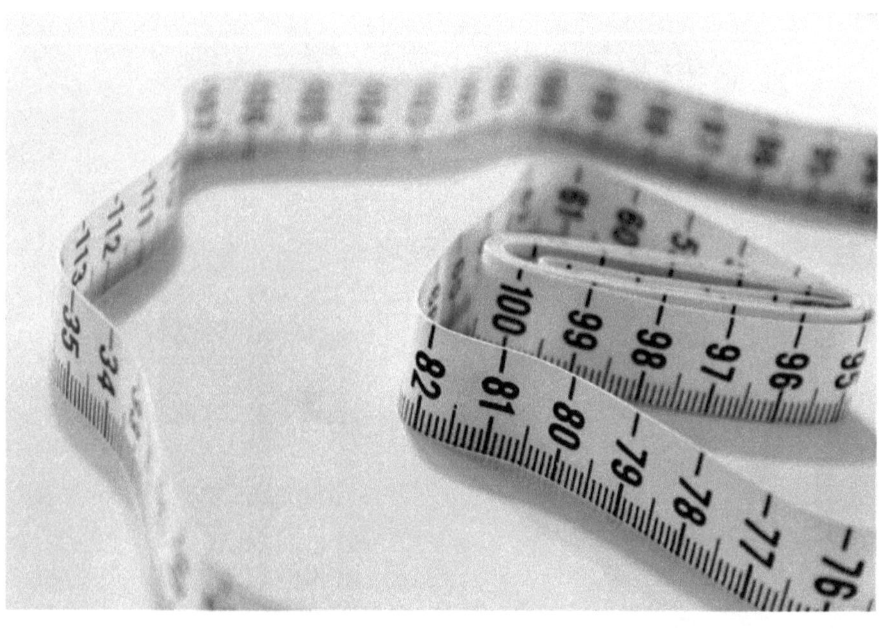

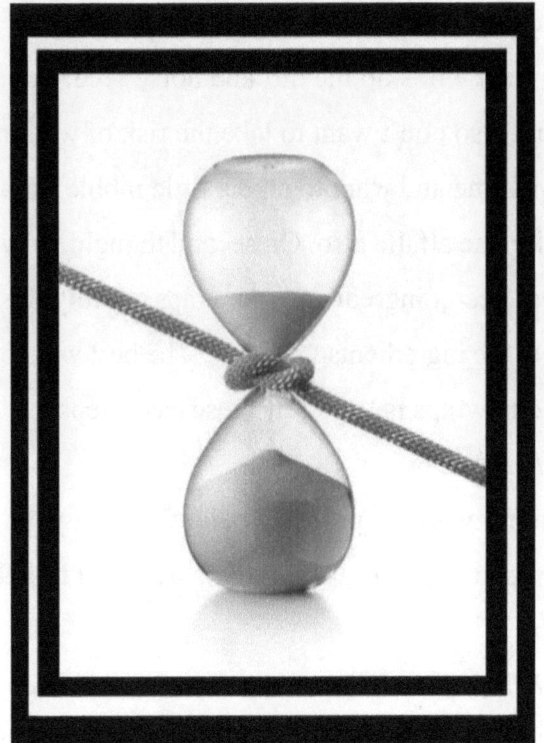

Chapter 8

Wrap it UP!

Body wraps are a surefire approach to free undesirable inches. They also can nourish and hydrate your skin at the same time, tighten your skin while decreasing cellulite. Also, body wraps have a bonus of removing toxins from your body. Body wrap ingredients usually contain clay, aloe, seaweed, and sea salt. However, some body-wraps also include "secret ingredients" such as dandelion root and alfalfa leaves, horse feed, dirt, aloe, seaweed, and sea salt. I like the idea of many of the "secret ingredients," but I will skip the dirt and horse feed. I don't like those ingredients and also don't want to take the risk of walking by a horse that might smell me and want to take a little nibble for a snack. So, I guess I will skip the alfalfa also. On second thought, why not just skip the overpriced "secret ingredient" spa wraps entirely. Instead, make a wrap with only the ingredients you want. The best way to get the most out of your body wraps is to follow these easy steps.

Step 1: Hydrate

Hydrating yourself properly before getting your wrap cannot be stressed enough. Hydration is essential to help flush your system.

Step 2 Exfoliate the area you are about to wrap

Use a dry brush to remove dead skin or better use the dry brush then try one of the body scrubs in Chapter 5 like the Mocha Scrub. Another option is to have microdermabrasion done on the specific area, then wait a day to do the wrap.

Step 3: Wrap it UP!

Using one of the recipes in this chapter, apply a thin layer of the mixture to your skin on the area you want to wrap. Focusing on the area, you want to lose inches, reduce the appearance of cellulite or firm up. Remember a little goes a long way. You do not need to apply a large amount because these mixtures are very effective. Only apply one section at a time then wrap with plastic wrap and elastic bands. For best results, it is recommended to use both for plastic wrap and bands. After you have one area wrapped and secure move to your next area and repeated the process until you have all the areas you want to be wrapped covered. Warning: DO NOT wrap too tightly! You want to feel compression but not be uncomfortable in any way. You need to be able to breathe and always continue to have proper circulation throughout your body.

Step 4: Relax and Sweat It Out

Put on your robe and cover yourself with a warm blanket or heating pad. If you have a portable sauna, this would be a great time to use it if you are not home alone. You want to make sure you are nice and warm, so your body starts to sweat.

Step 5: Unwrap and Cleanse

After about 30 minutes to an hour, it is time to begin unwrapping yourself. After you have entirely unwrapped yourself, it is time to take a room temperature shower to cleanse your skin.

Step 6: Moisturize

At this time, your body will absorb products for optimum results. Please do not skip this step and take time to moisturize your body emphasizing on the wrapped area. If you were treating for stretch marks, this is the perfect time to apply your stretch mark cream.

Step 7: Fight Fat with Water

Drinking water makes your skin glow, and it can help you with weight loss. Drinking an 8-ounce bottle of water with each meal and one to sip on throughout the day will achieve a proper fluid intake for the day.

Step 8: Eat Healthy & Exercise

If you think you can celebrate with double cheeseburgers and a large order of fries, because you lost a few inches, think again. You need to eat healthily and exercise if you want to maintain or possibly improve the results you have just gotten.

Step 9: Stay Consistent

No matter how perfect you think you look now, you need to continue getting consistent body wrapping. Make wraps a part of your bi-weekly beauty routine and stick to it for permanent results.

Step 10: Don't Overdo It

Take it easy, have fun, and remember that it's a slow and gradual process. So, don't expect overnight results. I have never understood why the inches and weight goes on so very quickly but seem to take forever to lose.

Super Skin Body Wraps

I am sure by now; you are ready to get started wrapping away! Here are 5 DIY body wraps remember just as with everything else in this book, please let your imagination go until you create the wrap that is just right for you. Who's to say you may like the horse feed which wasn't right for me. These DIY body wraps are meant to be fun and serve as a good excuse for you to get some relaxing downtime. Remember to stay hydrated while doing your wrap. Before and after wrap measurements will show you how well the wrap worked for you.

Shrinky Wrap

Ingredients:

2 cups Green Tea

2 tablespoons Cayenne Powder

2 tablespoons Ginger Powder

1 cup Bentonite Clay Powder

1 drop Juniper Essential Oil

1 drop Cypress Essential Oil

1 drop Atlas Cedarwood Essential Oil

Directions:

Using a plastic bowl mix all ingredients to form a mud-like paste. Do not use any metal because it might react to the clay and draw traces of the metal. Follow the directions for the body wrap procedure described above.

Vicks Under Wraps

With just three simple ingredients, this is a quick mix for wrappers that want a little boost. Vicks VapoRub has been reported to help with congestions, weight loss, cellulite, tennis elbow, relieve sore muscle pain, reduce eczema, and stretch marks.

Ingredients:

1 six-ounce jar Vicks VapoRub

6 drops Eucalyptus Oil

1/4 cup Monoi Oil

Directions:

Mix all ingredients till well blended and massage on your body area that will be wrapped. Wrap yourself in plastic, followed by bandages. Put on your robe and wrap yourself in a warm blanket or possibly with a heating pad and relax for one hour.

Cellulite Under Wrap

Seaweed and clay both act as powerful ingredients in battling cellulite, shifting inches, and rejuvenating your body. Here's how you create one of the most effective wraps for cellulite:

Ingredients:

1 cup Seaweed Powder

3 tablespoons Monoi Oil

2 cups Warm Coffee

1 drop each Essential Oil (Rosemary, Juniper, and Fennel)

Directions:

Mix all the body wrap ingredients to form a mud-like consistency. Stand in your shower, on some newspapers or a large towel to minimize the mess. Start by smearing the paste all over the lower half of your body, followed by the upper half. Follow the directions for the body wrap procedure described above.

Mocha Cellulite Power Paste

Make a paste of equal amounts of coffee grounds and Sea Clay. Rub in circular motions, wrap your body, and leave on for 20 minutes. Rinse with warm water.

Wrap it Up

Ingredients:

2 cups Monoi Oil

6 drops of Grapefruit Essential Oil

2 drops each Vitamin E and A

2 drops each Wintergreen, Lavender, and Fennel Oil

Directions:

Mix all oils and pour into a spray bottle. Spray all over your skin and wrap in plastic then bandages. Stay warm area for an hour then shower with warm water.

That's a Wrap

Ingredients:

1 cup Epsom Salt

4 cups warm Chamomile Herbal Tea

4 tablespoons Monoi Oil

4 drops of Eucalyptus Essential Oil

Directions:

Mix warm tea and Epsom salt then soak wrapping bands or an old sheet in the solution. Mix oils and massage on your body. Wrap yourself in the warm sheet or bands, followed by a plastic wrap, to keep it all nicely packed for proper sweating. Put on your robe and wrap yourself in a warm blanket, possibly with a heating pad and relax for one hour. Remove all wraps then shower.

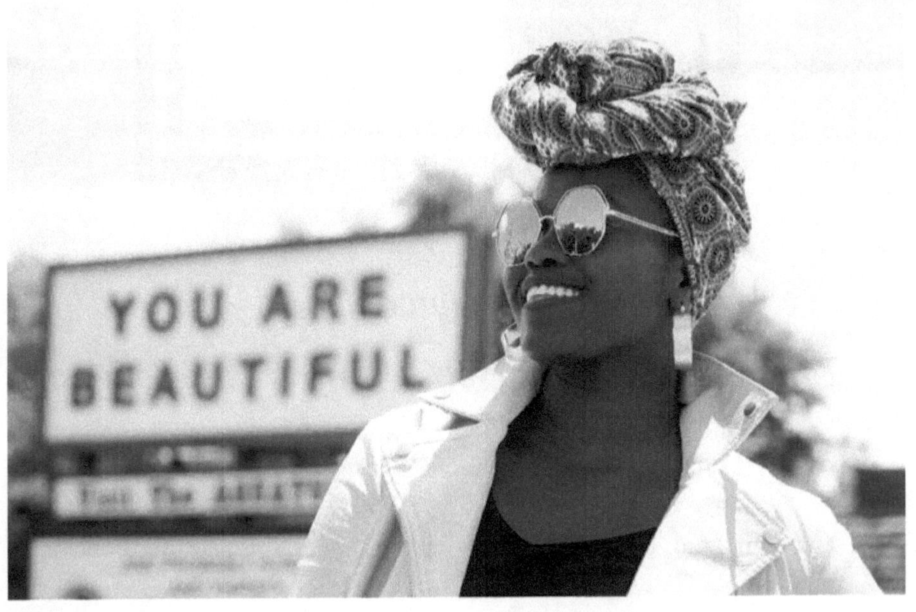
YOU ARE
BEAUTIFUL

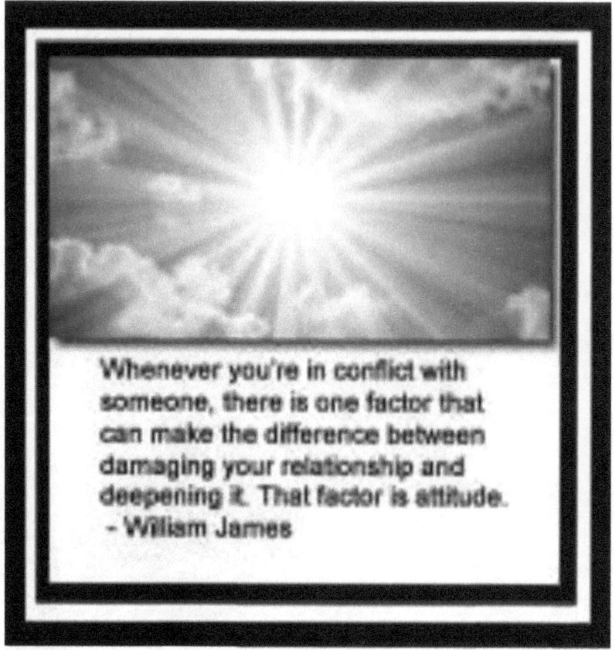

Chapter 9

Taking Care of Yourself Changes Your Outlook on Life

Latica Mirjanic, MA Psych contributed this chapter to the book.

[Latica Mirjanic has helped me for many years servings as one of the professional therapists assisting with the Divorced and Scared NO More book series and website. She is currently assisting the DASNM community on Facebook at Divorced and Scared NO More, Google Plus and Twitter @Divorced_Scared. In addition to helping me and my various fans around the world, Laticia takes care of her patients from various location through her website, UpperDeckSelf-Help.com. She is not only my friend but also my right-hand woman! I could not accomplish all I do without her help. Because I believe true beauty comes from within I felt it only fitting to have Latica weigh in and give her thoughts on the subject.]

Meeting Martha

Meet Martha. She's 47 years old. Has two kids still in school. She works like crazy, hates her boss, doesn't find a great interest in her job, helps her husband with his business, takes care of her parents all while she volunteers in her community once a week. Although Martha once read, she should practice gratitude; she can't help but feel exhausted when she wakes up every morning. It's been such a long time since she spent some time with her girlfriends. Her kids think she's a super-mom. She can do everything and make it seem like a breeze. The problem is that Martha feels strong headaches every weekend. Instead of relaxing, she suffers and hopes this new painkiller will get her some relief. When her husband points out that she should relax more, she knows that she just doesn't have the time. Take a moment to mentally write down your Martha story based on your obligations and your life. Is "all of it" causing problems for you already? Have you ever decided to do something about it? Maybe you are like Martha. Maybe for you, it is impossible to find the time. Do you sometimes read how you should be doing meditation, mindfulness or a plain early morning run and think that it sounds nice but just doesn't work in real life?

How your drive works

Making a decision to take good care of yourself means that you have an intention to recover from whatever circumstances that are putting pressure on you. In psychological counseling, we often observe two broad ways of human functioning. One has the element of destruction and alienation, and the other holds elements of creation and cooperation. We, as human beings, need both of them to survive.

In everyday life, escaping death is such a strong instinct that it often consumes our entire perception. Just observe how negatively oriented are news all over TV and the internet. You don't even have to go that far into the environment. Just observe your daily thoughts and actions. Do you do things to create something or not to lose something?

The difference is great. When you work at a job not to lose the apartment or when you get stuck in a relationship just to escape loneliness, you predominantly take action based on your bad feelings. In contrast, when you strive for easy and stress-free moments or work on tasks based on your ambition, your actions are a reflection of feelings such as relief or excitement. The secret behind these positive feelings is that it allows you to have a choice in your actions. You also have the freedom to do more because you have more resources to draw upon. You don't feel as exhausted.

Little contrasts like these tend to add up over time, and they really do reflect on your health. In order to identify which approach governs your life, take an honest look at where your perception stands. How often do you focus on your strengths and solving problems? Is your mind consumed by your illness, the past, future problems, or do you focus on simple, wonderful life events and look forward to the future?

Are you on your way to illness?

If I ask you where you want your life to go or please state what you would do more of if you could, you would probably give me some positive boxes to check along with a positive, ambitious plan.

But, if I ask you how you treat yourself in your everyday life, would you give me the same positive outlook or would you pull up all of the excuses and life circumstances that are preventing you from a healthy lifestyle? I'm not talking about sitting down in front of a TV every night. I'm talking about maintaining your physical, spiritual, and emotional health in real life.

In essence, self-care urges you to live healthy by eating healthy, exercising, making sure you get enough sleep, spend time outdoors, see friends, enjoy simple things and do something enjoyable every day like a hobby, spend time with pets, etc. You also need to find ways to manage stress, find ways to relax by meditating, doing yoga, and spending time in nature.

If this sounds like an impossible to-do list, you are not alone. A lot of people tend to ask why they can't just be lazy. The broad answer to that question is that you will slowly lose resilience, your ability to be less affected by other people or circumstances, and your ability to recover from illness.

This will make you more susceptible to diseases, unhealthy relationships, burnout, anxiety, depression, and diminished well-being. One of the biggest problems with this is that most people ignore their breaking point, even when they know what their breaking point is (e.g., fatigue, being rude, agitated by others, clumsy, etc.). When your duties and demands from the environment are more important than you, and your ability to take really good care of yourself, the quality and quantity of successfully executing those duties will diminish exponentially.

The Value of Self-Care

What is most important, you will not recover until you establish a balance between your personal needs and your workload or demands other people put on you. Even taking a short mental break will do wonders for your emotional capacity, focus, and sharpness. The value of inserting self-care into your everyday life lies in the fact that you will have regular breaks from life, and in that way, you will prevent yourself from reaching a breaking point. You can afford a quiet moment without distractions even if it's just a few moments every day.

Another great and valuable resource might be just spending time with people that are supportive, understanding, and inspirational to you.

These people make us feel relaxed and let us forget our problems and anxieties. And this helps us in the same way as a financial or any other form of help does. The problem is that people tend to sacrifice so much in-person social contact for other things. Mind that virtual socializing still has to demonstrate the same immediate effect.

Needless to say, that if people close to you are poisonous and toxic, you will not benefit from such relationships. With those types of relationships, you need to practice saying no or at least establish healthy boundaries. Nothing will work out if you suffer daily and trust me, with this sort of relationships you do suffer greatly. If you are repeatedly left by feeling bad, exhausted, let down or used, things won't miraculously improve.

How Self-Care Improves Our Outlook on Life

Knowing that you devote time and energy to yourself and that you can count on yourself for fulfilling your needs for rest or fun, means to practice self-love. If you make an effort to allow yourself leisure and activities that bring you joy, excitement, or a sense of relief, you will actively be storing food for harsh winters to come. Self-love can produce positive feelings at will, even in stressful situations, which improves your resilience, self-esteem, and confidence. So, to face life head-on almost every day, you need to establish a self-care routine in your everyday life.

Self-care has the power to strengthen our core because it has been proven to be related to a greater sense of well-being, which, in its essence, is emotional balance and perceived satisfaction with life. Be stronger healthier, build better relationships, and feel more hopeful about the future. It's optimism that makes them reach for higher goals and ensures they have more drive to achieve those goals, which in turn enhances their well-being. Just a little bit of self-care can set this positive spiral into motion.

Yes, that's right. Getting enough sleep, working out, maintaining a healthy weight, and eating nutritious foods, taking a break, pampering yourself to a massage and soothing DIY treatments can do all that. That is why it pays off to put some effort into incorporating self-care into your schedule. There can't be any excuses, because just 7 minutes of working out have positive effects on our brain.

Building A Happy Life

With self-care routines, you'll be faster in accomplishing tasks, and you will work more effectively because you won't break, become exhausted, give up and live a life of misery, stress, and self-pity. You will allow yourself to be happy and confident, be autonomous, attentive, emotionally balanced, and have good relationships at work and in your personal life.

Most of all, you will be better equipped to survive and recover from rejection, humiliation, conflict, or a negative person because you will be more resilient. This is often referred to as self-regulation, and it allows you to carry on with confidence and a positive outlook.

One of the tricks to emotional self-care is to acknowledge your feelings by saying how you feel to yourself. Taking a moment to observe whether you are angry, rejected, annoyed, tired, or sad can benefit you because it frees your mind to do other things. When the emotions are said, they come out of your psyche and don't creep in when you're trying to do other things.

I know it's easy to say leave your work problems when you shut the door to your office, but with practice, this will do miracles. Imagine coming home to a soothing bath without any distractions, your very own personal mental spa at will. You really can slow down. You don't need to solve all the problems in every minute of the day. Nothing will escape until the next morning.

To get yourself started, practice something that brings joy into your life. Some people read, some hike, some play video games, some take long baths. Find your hobby and take some time out of your busy schedule to make yourself happy and carefree. You will come back to that schedule recharged and motivated.

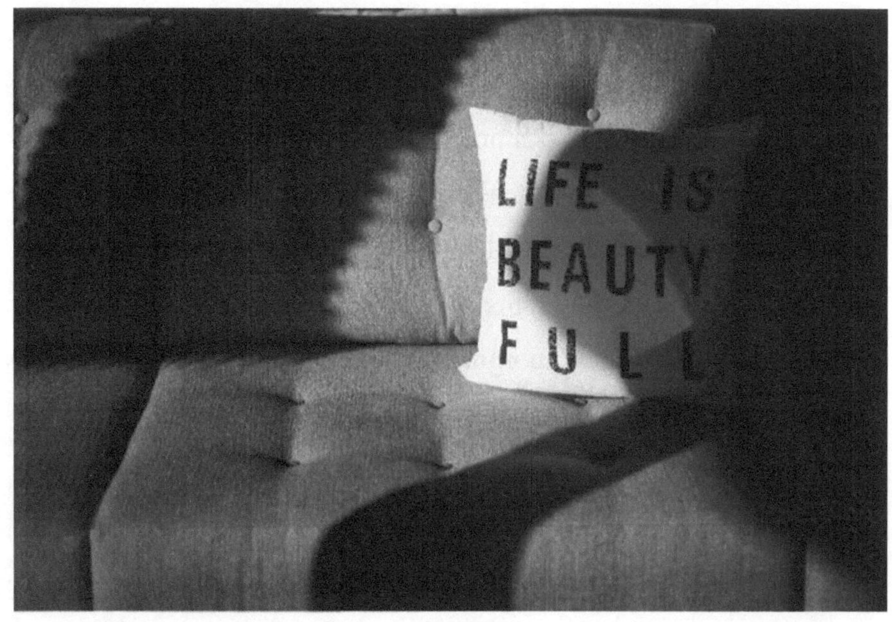
LIFE IS
BEAUTY
FULL

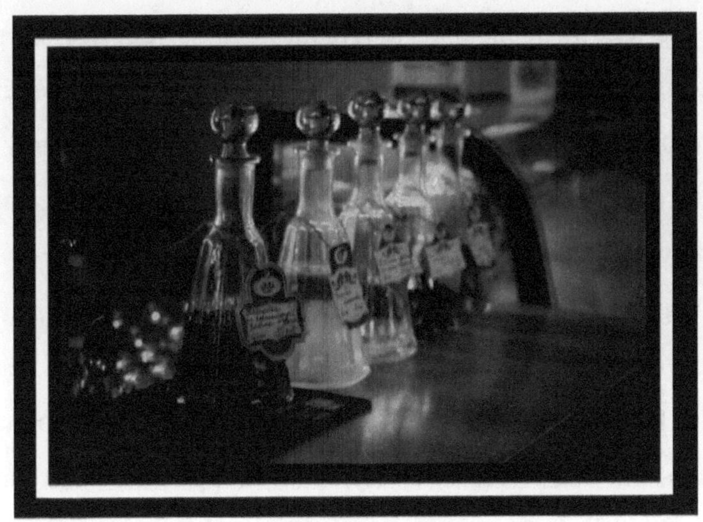

Chapter 10

Next Step – Knowledge, Imagination, and Creativity

These are just a few ideas that are noninvasive anti-aging treatments and a few easy ways of making your beauty treatments at home. The best part of doing your homemade items is that they don't come with any undesirable ingredients that can cause side effects. Before you grab your wallet and rush to buy over the counter items, check out these homemade recipes and use your imagination, adding your "secret ingredient." The products you make will only have what you like in them, and they will save you money!

No longer tell people your age when they ask instead respond "I am over _____" Let them use their judgment to guess your age. I am very proud to say I am over 50 and pleasantly pleased when people respond they are surprised by that. Before you ask, I won't tell you how many numbers over 50 I am. In a year or so I will start answering that question with "I am over 55"!

Knowledge is power, arm yourself with as much as you can, while starting your journey into a more balanced, spiritual, and healthier lifestyle. Collect as much information as you can about toxins and chemicals that lurk in our everyday beauty supplies that surround our store shelves. Before you agree to invasive beauty treatments that have many potential side effects and can take weeks to heal, consider trying some of the noninvasive beauty treatments available to you now. Let your imagination and creativity run wild and free with your newfound knowledge create your own "Precious" beauty products as unique as you are. Make a change today to use natural and noninvasive treatments for a younger, healthier you!

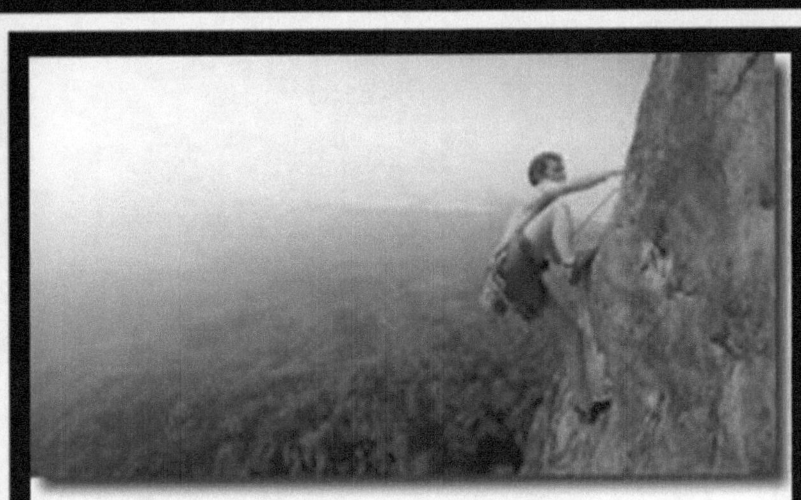

Courage doesn't always roar.
Sometimes courage is the quiet voice
at the end of the day saying, "I will try
again tomorrow."
- Mary Anne Radmacher

About the Author

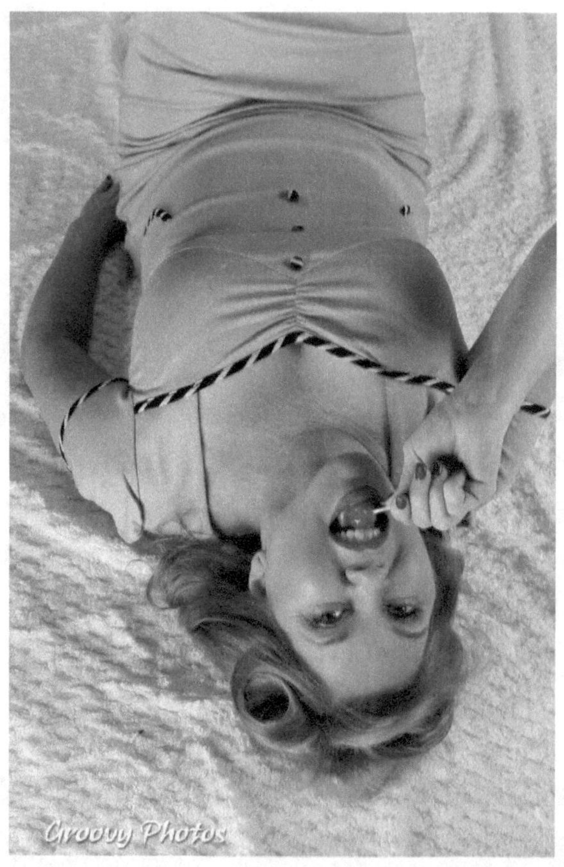

Tammy Asher, aka Tasher, is the author of the Divorced and Scared NO More Series. Emotional Support for the Newly Divorced, Practical Advice for the Newly Divorced and Dating After Divorce— From Lemons to Zesty Lemon Sorbet are all available on Amazon.com. Tasher was divorced on her 26th wedding anniversary, and she embarked on a new life. Her marriage was broken all to pieces; she was not going to let the divorce break her. Tasher quickly discovered that single life was very different from all those years ago. One case in point is dating; there was not an internet back then, and cell phones didn't exist. Like many, she initially was scared but being a smart businessperson; she set up a plan of how to date yet continue to keep her and family safe.

Tasher has dyslexia yet always enjoyed writing and decided to share with others the things she learned while rebuilding her life. The launch of Divorced and Scared No More.com was November 2012 and quickly received a worldwide following. As she started sharing her experiences, others in-turn shared some of their stories. The intent of the site was for people to share without fear of reprisals. The website logos inspiration was a set of broken pilot wings (her ex-husband is a pilot). The DASNM website has been shut down, but the Facebook page and Twitter are still available for people to access.

Tasher lives in Texan and a mother of three adult children, a proud Grammy to three grandchildren and two step-grandchildren. You can follow Tasher or on Facebook at Divorced and Scared NO More, Google Plus and Twitter @Divorced_Scared. You can also see her on YouTube at T asher discussing "What is Forgiveness," "The Internet, Your Ex, and the Legal System" and "How Do I Know When I am Ready to Date."

About the Contributor

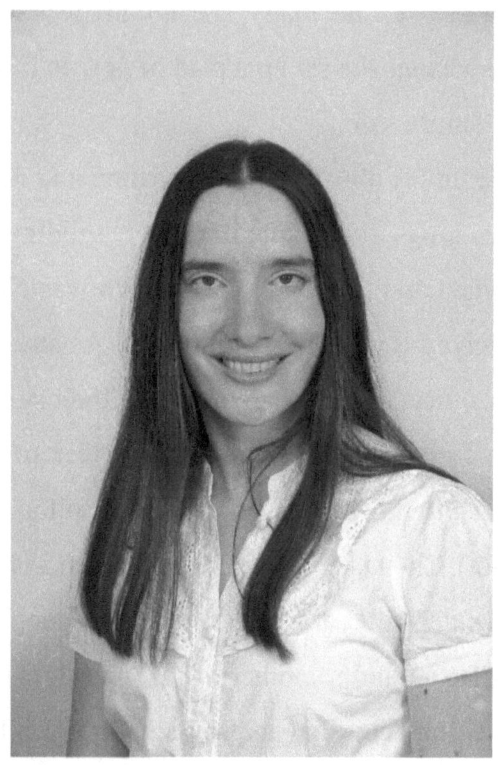

Latica Mirjanic, MA Psych

LATICA MIRJANIC is a psychologist (MA) from Zagreb, Croatia, the EU. She's an expert in the field of positive psychology, which is founded on the belief that people want to lead meaningful and fulfilling lives and to enhance their experiences of love, work, and play. She has helped countless people transform their personal and professional lives in more than eight years of experience in psychological counseling, research, and project implementation.

She came up with the idea of "upper deck self-help" and "wear the new you" concepts after seeing how people who get more support for their situation get faster and better results. She aims to make support practical and manageable with an emphasis on the empowerment of people to take responsibility and achieve change.

In her work, she's witnessed countless times that a person can preserve and strengthen their mental and consequently physical health and that it's always possible to live a more balanced and successful life. Since 2012 has been servings as one of the professional therapists assisting with the Divorced and Scared NO More book series and website.

She is currently still assisting with the DASNM community on Facebook at DivorcedAndScaredNoMore, and Twitter @Divorced_Scared.Her other great passion is creating stories for children. She finds inspiration in her everyday life and surrounding. A child's world is all fun and magic, and so are her stories.

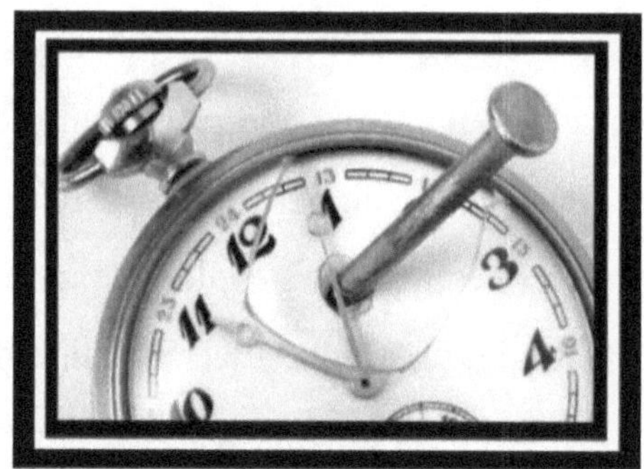

Contact and Links

Tammy Asher aka Tasher

Email hbty18@gmail.com

Facebook DivorcedAndScaredNoMore

Twitter @Divorced_Scared

YouTube T asher

Latica Mirjanic, MA Psych

Email wearthenewyou@gmail.com or

mailto:upperdeckselfhelp@gmail.com

Website UpperDeckSelfHelp.com

Sandraspeed Book Formatting Expert

Email sandraspeed@writeme.com

All Graphics courtesy of

Divorced and Scared NO More website or books, Unsplash.com,

Stockfreeimages.com, Istockphoto.com and Freephotos

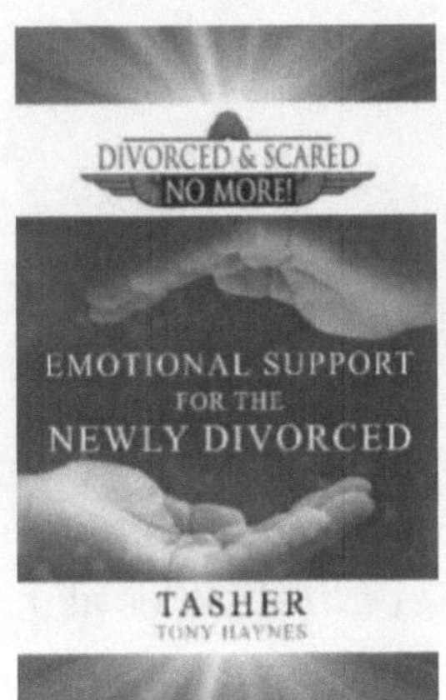
DIVORCED & SCARED
NO MORE!
EMOTIONAL SUPPORT
FOR THE
NEWLY DIVORCED
TASHER
TONY HAYNES

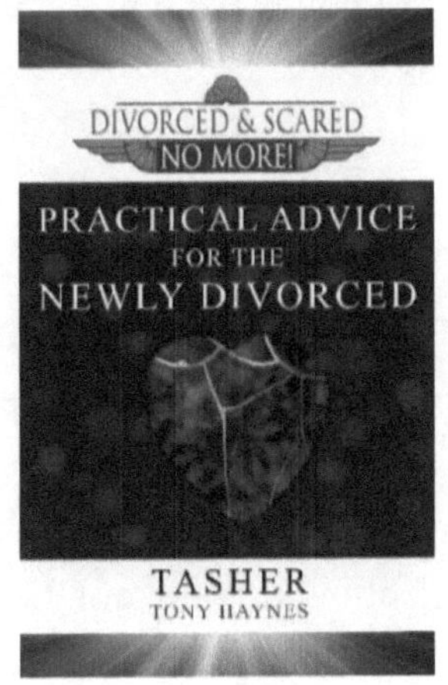
DIVORCED & SCARED
NO MORE!
PRACTICAL ADVICE
FOR THE
NEWLY DIVORCED
TASHER
TONY HAYNES

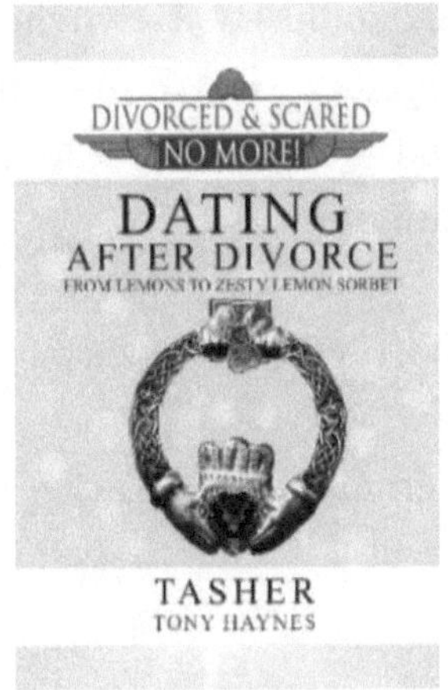
DIVORCED & SCARED
NO MORE!
DATING
AFTER DIVORCE
FROM LEMONS TO ZESTY LEMON SORBET
TASHER
TONY HAYNES

✳✳✳

Dear Reader,

Thank you, so much for buying my book Holdin' Back the Years. I want to thank you for being one of our readers!

I hope that you've enjoyed reading the book. I want to make sure this book provided you with the value you needed. Hopefully, you have learned at least one or two tips that will help you feel better about yourself while saving you money. I also believe many of the suggestions in this book are better for you than many of the expensive store-bought similar items.

If you have ANY issues or feedback, please email me at HBTY18@gmail.com. The only way I can improve the books are with your help. I would be honored to get your honest opinion of this book in the review section where you purchased the book!

Thank you again for ordering my book. I truly appreciate your business. Hopefully, the book helped not be afraid to create your unique version of Hocus Pocus. Maybe you have become like Samantha in Bewitched or gotten a little group of Golden Girls together to have fun with the ideas within this book. Not only to feel and look better but to also hold back those pesky numbers that keep climbing.

Wishing you the best,

Tammy Asher aka Tasher

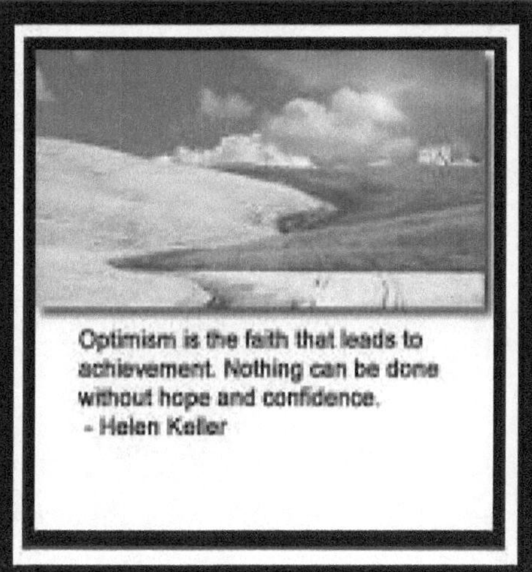
Optimism is the faith that leads to
achievement. Nothing can be done
without hope and confidence.
- Helen Keller

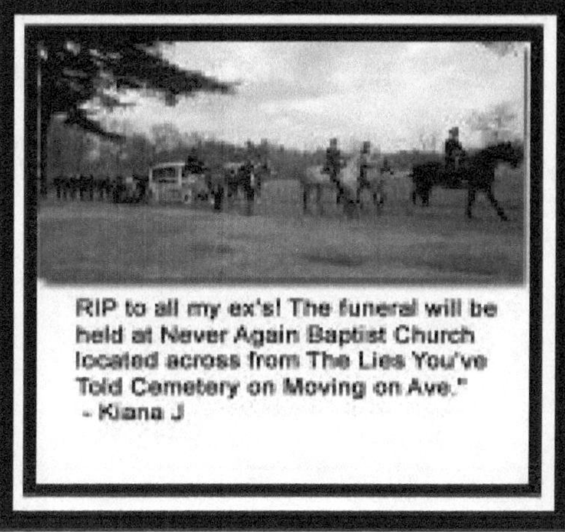
RIP to all my ex's! The funeral will be
held at Never Again Baptist Church
located across from The Lies You've
Told Cemetery on Moving on Ave."
- Kiana J

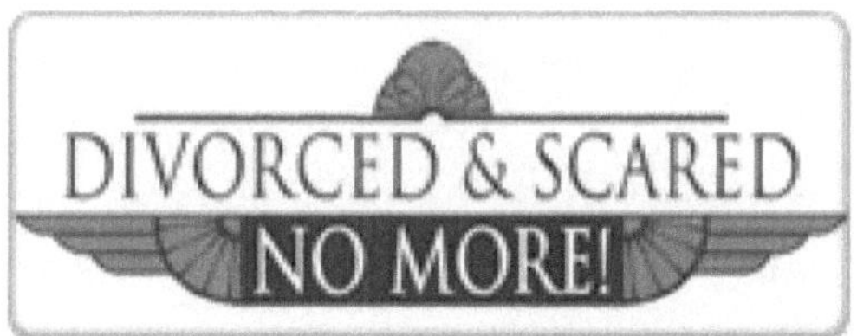
DIVORCED & SCARED
NO MORE!